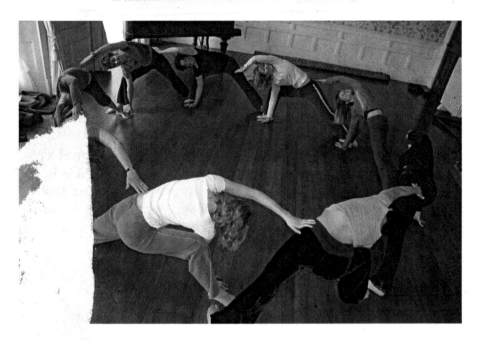

OGA. HOW AND WHY IT WORKS

Examination of the Reason for the Effectiveness of Yoga as a
System of Physical, Mental and Spiritual Cultivation

Andy Thomas

D1347913

Published 2009 by arima publishing

www.arimapublishing.com

ISBN 978 1 84549 367 7

© Andy Thomas 2009

Printed and bound in the United Kingdom

Typeset in Garamond 12/14

Swirl is an imprint of arima publishing.

arima publishing
ASK House, Northgate Avenue
Bury St Edmunds, Suffolk IP32 6BB
t: (+44) 01284 700321

www.arimapublishing.com

CONTENTS

PREFACE

While preparing for a brand new course which I conceived around the middle of 2007, I found numerous fascinating references to how human disease and dysfunction should be treated by the physician, whatever his discipline and inclination. These appeared in a wide variety of books most of which I acquired during my own training 25 years ago. These references were what I would describe as tantalisingly close to the position that we in yoga and fmm would take. Because of this closeness I have decided, just before finalising this book for publication, to include all these references. It felt to me as if they really were intended to be read and inwardly digested by those learning the disciplines of fmm and yoga. I leave you to judge the accuracy of that thought. It is probable that I read them all that time ago and that they meant little then.

Here is the first, though they are presented in no particular order, each having its own message and each having its own prominence!!
This is from Applied Anatomy 1903, an osteopathic text book.

"Disease, in the average case, is due to a disturbance of structure. Even in cases of disease resulting from abuse, there is often found some structural change. In all diseases, whether from abuse or other causes, there are to be found structural changes, peculiar to the disease. These structural changes are, in a general way, called lesions.

Lesions, therefore, may be ligamentous, muscular, visceral or bony."

Clarke, M.E., 1903 *Applied Anatomy*
Tunbridge Wells. Maidstone College of Osteopathy

The case continues to be made along the same lines and the writer claims that the bony lesion—or problem—affects the way the bones interact, impairing function. He says that anything which disturbs the way the joint moves can be classed as a bony problem and that this will be the result of ligamentous shortening, muscle contracture-(note the use of the term contracture which is the same term as used by medical professionals) or perhaps even bony outgrowths. But an inflammatory deposit will have the same result and this can be caused by the most minute of injuries, these setting up exudates which splint the area and begin the process of mobility restriction. The statement is that this is the primary cause of all disorders.

The writer continues to make the case for all diseases and dysfunctions to have their true origin here and he says that physical culture is not a substitute for osteopathic treatment since the movements of the spine take place in the normal parts, while the place of injury is not moved at all. To reduce such a lesion, passive movement must be directed to the injured joint. By doing this the function is temporarily restored, the circulation through the part bettered and absorption of the deposits begins. This is followed by restoration of function of the joint and the adjacent tissues. Such conditions predispose to visceral disease.

In lesions of the spinal column there is in practically all cases a deposit around the joint and a thinning of the intervertebral disc. The end result to be worked for, in the treatment of the spine, is to restore normal function—that is to say, normal movement- to the spinal articulations. This can be achieved by adjusting the surfaces and by stretching the inflamed tissues around the injured joint. The most significant cause of bony lesions producing disease is pressure on nerves, vessels and other tissues, principally at the intervertebral foramina from where blood vessels and nerve roots emerge The pressure is from the displaced bone or is a result of the inflammatory deposits around the injured joint. On account of this, the nerve connections between the spinal cord and the rest of the body are interrupted, the blood vessels supplying and draining the spinal cord compressed, the lymphatic vessels impaired and as a result of this, the nutrition of the cord disturbed, the originating impulses interfered with as well as the transmission of them. Normal circulation to the spinal cord is essential to proper functioning of it.

The above paraphrasing sets out unequivocally the process of disorder. As someone involved in yoga and therapy you may see that it is not quite followed to the end of the origin of things—that the soft tissue is what shrinks to create the opportunity for the lesion to be created. There will be more discussion on this issue.

We move now to another book.
"The examination and treatment of any peripheral joint (this means shoulder, knee etc) inevitably means a consideration of the anatomy of that joint together with its pathological condition. As far as spinal lesions

are concerned, however, this has not been general practice and the tendency to treat solely signs and symptoms without due regard to the clinical diagnosis is fraught with danger."

Oliver, J and Middleditch, A.1991 *Functional Anatomy of the Spine*
Oxford, Butterworth and Heinemann

The writers make this point clearly—it is certainly not general practice and they state that:

"The spine is often regarded as being far too complex to attempt to form a specific diagnosis unless the problem is obvious---- the prolapsed intervertebral disc with nerve root involvement is the classic case, they state. To make an intelligent diagnosis saves the patient time and trouble, they say, with signs and symptoms not in any way being disregarded but the interpretation of them is clearer. An accurate diagnosis will also prevent over –zealous manipulation of joints in the presence of, for example, instability or vertebral artery disease they add. If only it were so—it is not my experience. Many of the patients and yoga students I receive have despaired at the lack of understanding from, typically, physiotherapists."

There are many statements that could with value be quoted----and this book is absolutely typical of those written by physiotherapists. There are many references to accurate diagnosis and appropriate treatment. But first, read this from the very famous Dr James Cyriax, one time consultant orthopaedic surgeon at St. Thomas's Hospital in London.

This appears in his text book called The Textbook of Orthopaedic Medicine and is in Chapter 1 entitled Logical Treatment.

"When I was a medical student I read and re-read Bertrand Russell "Sceptical Essays". He put forward convincing arguments in favour of reason as against mere custom as a basis for conduct and set out the radical changes that would follow the application of this logical code to ordinary every day life. Even so, though the unarguable concepts put before the reader are simple, *much of today's physiotherapy would be revolutionised if they were acted upon.*

Cyriax, J 1982 *Textbook of Orthopaedic Medicine*
London .Bailliere Tindall

Here Cyriax slates physiotherapists—as he does osteopaths and chiropractors!!- stating that his work is based on the simple principles – that pain arises from a lesion and treatment must reach the lesion. He claims that these are childishly simple but violated daily. He goes on to say that heat and ice are regularly applied when all should know that the effect is entirely superficial and cannot reach the lesion. The physiotherapist will not even make an effort to manipulate the piece of displaced intervertebral disc out of the way even when the diagnosis is obvious.

Any reader would smile superciliously if he heard that in Asia the devils were driven out of a man's painful back by the application of hot dung; but here today many doctors and physios are not ashamed to give infrared in lumbago. What is the difference? This is his closing remark on the subject!!

During my own osteopathic training in the early 80's I attended several of the courses offered to physios and run by the good doctor when he was still alive. He was utterly scathing about doctors, physios, osteopaths and chiropractors in their attempts to treat people. There are always numerous pages in all his books devoted to slating all practitioners for not behaving logically. Still, however, he did not make any connection with fascial contracture being the motor of all musculoskeletal conditions. But there is one person who is in no doubt. Ida Rolf who "invented "Rolfing. In the late 80's I met an American Rolfer who taught me, along with a group of osteopaths, how to Rolf a human body following a postural assessment. Much of what I learned is incorporated in Full Movement Method, which I chose to patent just as did Feldenkrais, Alexander, Rolf and Bowen have done for much the same reasons. Not to keep to ourselves but to attempt to protect the purity of what has evolved in our hands.

Here is Dr Ida Rolf during her pioneering days. These are snippets from her book written near the end of her life and about her work which have been written by those who worked with her.

"She had always investigated what was new and was never afraid to take what she learned and use it. She already knew a fair amount about osteopathy and homoeopathy and yoga. All these she investigated out of concern for her own health which had been affected by being kicked by a horse. She visited an osteopath at the time and got well as a result". She continues;

"Osteopathic treatment changes the way the bones of the body relate to one another, freeing obstructions between joints and thereby improving well-being. Similarly, Rolfing seeks to enhance function by changing structure, but it differs from osteopathy in two important ways. As Rolfers, we see that bones are held in place by soft tissue—muscles, ligaments, tendons etc. If a muscle is chronically short, it will pull the attached bone out of balance.

Repositioning the bone is not enough; the individual muscle and allied tissue must be lengthened if the change is to be permanent. In addition, when the body is out of balance in one part, others are affected so it must be restored to normal balance.
Rolf, I 1960 *Ida Rolf Talks*. Colorado, Boulder Press.

All through the 1920's Ida belonged to a group of yoga practitioners who practised yoga asanas. When she was working with patients she first worked with the techniques of yoga, instructing through movement. Slowly she realised that the asanas did not always reach an active separation of joint surfaces and that something else was needed. She discovered mobilisation techniques that later evolved into what is now called Rolfing, by manually stretching tissues. Ida tried to teach her point of view to chiropractors and osteopaths but eventually realised that they just wanted the techniques and did not wish to take the philosophy with it, nor to see the human as a complete organism. She then decided to pass on the body of knowledge to body workers who were then treated as lay people. This led to the establishment of the Rolf Institute which exists today in Boulder, Colorado U.SA.

There will be many such references in later chapters. The reason for including this in a yoga work is, I sincerely hope, very obvious and not requiring explanation. If this is not clear yet I hope it will become so in later chapters.

Another book about yoga, you may say. Can another be justified? Is another really valuable? The process of yoga has been around for many thousands of years—surely everything that could be said has already been said?

My discovery over more than twenty two years of practising yoga and teaching it for over 17 of those years, is that ignorance abounds. Even amongst people who could be assumed to be "expert" (of course, we have a difficulty with this word before we start!!) there is much superficial understanding especially when there is a call for the student or sufferer needing guidance to be given specific instructions which will work. The person in pain or who has great difficulty in performing/perfecting a posture will be, most often, the seeker who is given spurious advice by those who do not really know. The reason for their not knowing is simple—real knowing comes from deep self-practise and not from training courses or books. It does not have an external source—so real "knowing" has to come from much observation of others as well as of self.

To the question often posed by the sufferer----"what should I do?" --the answer is usually "practise yoga" or practise more, and for greater time than you are currently doing or more intensively or add this particular posture or modify that particular posture. In the many workshops which I have led, even the most knowledgeable person has been obliged to reconsider his or her position in the light of the evidence produced in the workshop situation. There is much "information" that has come from a pool that is not the genuine pool of knowledge from which the data in this book is taken. The real source of knowledge for the ancient yogis-the "rishis" or seers—was deep introspection and consistent testing of "theory". The Pradipika and many of the modern books on yoga that are truthful, state that yoga must be verified by ones own practise. This means that the successful individual has understood the need for self-motivation to increase genuine knowledge. This strongly implies that the individual will not succeed unless there is this delving into the "own-mind pool". The pool of real knowledge cannot come in a book nor can it come from that class of teacher that has consistently created *limitations* for the students. The teacher who tells the class that the head stand should not be done or that the cobra is to be avoided if it involves neck extension, demonstrates a very deep and wide chasm in his knowledge. Prohibitions do not work for the benefit of the student and automatically prevent his/her from exploring the deep aspects of yoga, the real source of knowledge. There is an old saying in teaching generally—don't teach what you don't know. Of course it is easy to see how this could be applied to mathematics but less easy to see how it could be applied to yoga.

Is this book necessary? –we say yes, of course. Not because it is revolutionary but because it charts the ground explored by adventurous practitioners of the art, not only on their own personal journey but—probably more importantly—the learning that has gone with teaching thousands of people the art of yoga. Whilst all this learning has gone on for the students, the observers—we the teachers —have been computing (sometimes unconsciously but usually consciously), what has been happening in the body being viewed. The person in the class-everyone in the class but especially the one who is suffering—is the mobile laboratory in which we conduct all our experiments. Each person who submits themselves to any workshop in which we are the leaders, is automatically in our laboratory for examination. This is very much what we might call the Western model of analysis, not like the Eastern model of yoga in which the guru simply tells the students what to do and has no attachment to the outcome nor any interest in the obstacles within the students except in so far as the guru is able to tell the students to work harder at a particular posture.

This is not trying to reinvent anything. We accept that we are Westerners. We are not modifying yoga in any way. We are not saying anything that could be contentious for a genuine Eastern yogi since we have spent much time with experts. What we discovered on many occasions, however, was that the expert did not understand in the way the Western mind sometimes demands to know, how and why things occur as they do, It must be added, also, that there have been many thousands of patients in our clinics over nearly three decades of therapy and this we know to have produced unique knowledge. When added to the stock of unique knowledge of yoga it can be shown that the methods which we use to solve the problems of the sufferer WORK because we DO understand how it all works. Well—we cannot claim that we always get it right but for most of the time the students and sufferers get better just as 95% of our patients get better. This is so with treatment even when considering that the majority of patients have been elsewhere for treatment before attending our clinics and have not improved. This tends to show that modern practitioners of physical therapy (especially physiotherapists) also do not understand the fundamentals of WHY the human body malfunctions nor WHAT to do other than the application of their prescription of joint crunching or whatever formula they were given during training. Indeed, we would incline to the view that there has always been one group of people who fully understood how the body needed to be treated to make it well—this is those calling themselves yogis.!

The knowledge we give here is to aid your understanding of the process of yoga. Nothing we say will help you with the discipline needed to make a success of yoga, What we hope is that you will realise that, at a certain point, more of the same will just not work. This book, then, will set out the reasons for performing certain postures or other practices or the manner of performing such, with the justification based on deep understanding. Ultimately it is up to you if you want to make the knowledge work for you

Verify everything. Don't take what we say as the gospel truth! Remember that yoga is not for sheep!! Please recognise that this is what is said in Patanjali's Sutras.

We can only send our thanks to all those thousands of patients and students of yoga who have given such a huge chunk of themselves for analysis and without whom this knowledge would be supposition and conjecture. Which leads me to talk about conjecture. Much of what I write about the effects is from observation—of self, of students in my yoga classes, of "guinea pigs" in workshops, and student teachers during training and after training. Where a clearly " scientific " statement is made—perhaps about a certain percentage blood pressure reduction being the result of a certain posture, this is not my observation but reproduced from published data and comes from controlled trials of which many have been undertaken. Much of the printed research work appears in a journal printed in India known as Yoga Mimamsa and the prominent researchers would normally expect to have their finding published in this.

And I finish this section with a quotation from Swami Satyananda Sarawati printed in one of the Bihar School of Yoga occasional publications;

"Man today is sick because he thinks he is sick. Sickness and disease have no place in the life of a man who does not accept and tolerate self-limiting thoughts which are the real seeds of our myriad ailments. We stand hypnotized by the belief that disease and illness are our fate and destiny, rather than health and bliss which are truly our birthright and heritage. In order to emerge from our mass hypnosis and collective hysteria and to experience health, joy and creative fulfilment, we must make systematic application of yoga a daily occurrence."

INTRODUCTION

"The only things we learn from experience is that we learn nothing from experience. " George Bernard Shaw.

Despite thousands of years of history during which yoga has been practised in many countries of the world and by millions of people it is probably because it is primarily a system of spiritual development that it has escaped the glare of technical assessment to which systems of purely physical culture have been subjected. If you consider how much publicity has been given to Pilates, for example, over only a couple of decades, it is a wonder that yoga is still available. The reason for its still being popular is because only seekers actively seek it and the system itself somehow rejects those who have misunderstood its ways. This characteristic has most likely come about because what is attractive to the seeker is that yoga will satisfy everyone FOR LIFE whereas the other systems have a very limited shelf life. Those who come to yoga and do not wish to take it up seriously at home soon realise that they are in the company of the sort of people for whom this IS the great attraction. It then becomes obvious to anyone taking it up that change often comes very quickly. Participants in yoga commonly find the company of those whose company they normally espouse, no longer interesting! Yoga, then is primarily suited to the seekers after spiritual enlightenment. One of the great attractions of Pilates especially is that it is not spiritual and therefore one is not enticed to go into the deeply personal –the scariest part of all for most. Best avoid this because this is a hornets nest, a box of snakes—is a common thought, I suspect!!

This book has had a difficult birth---this is partly because the more I know the less interested I am in setting it down on paper Equally, the more knowledge acquired, the more students come forward to request learning so this in itself discourages writing since it has been shown in my method of teaching that much more learning takes place by gradual osmosis than by the taking of copious notes or the reading of many books. Using this method of teaching caused some consternation amongst students since all have been brought up in an educational system that espoused reading and writing at the expense of UNDERSTANDING. The reason for this ?—that passing examinations has been the prime target and that you need only short term memory for this—not much understanding is required.

It has been a tussle with motivation but this tussle was finally overcome largely as a result of requests from students who crave knowledge. All the attempts that I made to persuade students that note taking is wasted or that reading books on the subject is of very limited value amounted to very little effect ! It is also, I have to admit, stimulating to be challenged to write down knowledge which is a genuine expression of the old Greek origin of this word, knowledge—gnosis, which means to know from within!! Thus, this attempt follows that which the yogis proclaimed— knowledge comes from practice and self- assessment. The difficulty has been reconciling these two opposing facets, these two sides of the coin and as the presence of this book witnesses, the coin landed tails up - which means that I write it down!!!

I am always mightily grateful for the fact that yoga cannot be known other than by actually engaging in it thoroughly. There are no yoga experts as theorists—they have all done it and done it for a long time.

In my usual fashion, the book is set out in a logical manner. First the problem is set out—shall we call it the justification for the presence of the system of yoga and then with as much detail as I can muster, there is an explanation of the general reasons for the changes which follow the practising of yoga. This is followed by detailed exposition of the effect of the major postures.

The primary reason for the birth of yoga thousands of years ago has to be the "human condition" and what to do about it. The yogis of this time – we know them as the "rishis" which we understand to mean "seers" --- were looking inside themselves and observing what effect certain actions had. For example, how do you suppose anyone could come to discover that holding the chin down to the sternum while holding the breath, causes the heart to slow down? And why should this be of value? Attempts are made in this book to *justify* all that has been observed— perhaps *explain* is a better word since the presence of knowledge which we know actually *works* is sufficient justification.

There is no nonsense in yoga. What you see as the processes of yoga works for everyone provided the student of the system is prepared to follow those immortal words
    --practise with fortitude, perseverance and adventurously.

Everyone taught by me and everyone taught by students taught by me will improve their overall health by following the path of yoga.

What this book is not attempting is to be a manual of instruction, a how to practise yoga book. It is a book which sets out to show what effect yoga has. When I began learning yoga, it was difficult to find a yoga teacher —now there is one serving every village and every community. There is a great rising of interest in matters spiritual, probably in response to our spiritually deprived culture. But since most people come to yoga who are searching for better health, the physical benefits are focussed upon most strongly, since this is most straightforward to explain. If you seek a much greater depth of understanding of how to make the spiritual aspects of yoga work for you then I can recommend reading my second book which is called DEEP YOGA. This is all about the spiritual journey and how to make yoga effective.

I have not attempted to make this a book to cover all aspects. If you desire to know much more about the myofascial network, a most fascinating subject and which could take a lifetime to study fully!—then you can refer to the best book on the subject –Jobs Body—or you can read Message in the Body which is my first book and published as the book for the Shanti Yoga School members but which is freely available to any interested party. I have included a brief section on fascia.

PART I. THE HUMAN PROBLEMS AND HOW THEY OCCUR

1. The Human Condition.

This term, the human condition, turns up in all spiritual books. It generally refers to the mental condition—why someone is deeply unhappy. Why someone is depressed. Why someone cannot forgive a wrong done to them. Why does someone want to kill another.

Why does a young woman desperately fear becoming pregnant? We could fill the whole book with the individual expressions that I and my colleagues have heard from our patients. Just this small sample would fill this book and we have only treated a handful of people in comparison with the population. But the human condition is not just mental although I would always state my opinion that all disease and dysfunction has a mental origin. It must be obvious that the vast majority of doctors' consultations involve the patient in stating a physical symptom. Indeed, this is also the case for me and all my colleagues in physical therapy.

So-what is the **physical** human condition? Generally it can be summarised as a loss of functional quality. This demands explanation

Let us take the baby at a time when it is possible to see that it is fully mobile. It sleeps when it wishes and demands to be fed when it is hungry. No one would argue with this. Now try moving the limbs of the baby and observe how fluid is the movement, how soft and flexible it all feels. Now take the 5 year old as she starts school and go through the same movements as you did with the baby. For the most part you will find little difference but if you were to lie the child on her back and then stretch the hamstrings you would find that there is already some shortening. The baby state enables you to take the straight leg right to the point at which the knee touches the chin. This is the normal state. Now the 5 year old will not quite be capable of doing this and your attempt will be greeted with howls of protest. It is painful to attempt to stretch the hamstrings even on a 5 year old. So what has happened in that 4 years from the 1 year old baby to the five year old school child? The answer is simple—the hamstrings have begun to shorten—the myofascial network has begun to shrink as a result of one simple principle which will be spelled out in this book and the ignorance of which is almost universal in physical medicine and therapy of all kinds.

By the age of 15-17 there is already a serious loss in another department—the rib cage has begun to collapse as a result of poor posture—we will call it poor posture for the time being even though that is a grossly inadequate term - and the hamstrings are now so short that the youngster cannot bend even to touch his toes. This is especially so with boys involved in hard sports such as football and rugby. If you were to feel the muscles with your hands after a game of football or rugby you would be able, even without any formal training, to discern that they are hard!! They should not be like this at any age but especially not at such a tender age.

Now the teenager is preparing to go into the world of work which now will almost certainly be founded on computers. This will involve long periods sitting in a chair behind a desk and looking at a screen. This will cause further myofascial shrinkage of the abdominals and over- tensing of the posterior muscles of the spine. These will already show signs of contracture which can be a source of back pain. Most people in teenage will report some type of back pain at some time in their early life. Usually it is left unresolved, generally following a GP consultation in which there will be a string of platitudes about posture, too much tellie and so on. The boy or girl and the parent will be no wiser and no action will be taken. This is the pattern that we have observed in so many young people. The stresses of life will increase and the young person is subjected internally to an increase in unresolvable doses of adrenalin whilst at work. The rib cage depression is now so common that it would not be noticed in any company—but the function of the heart and all that goes with it, is seriously compromised.

Bring along, in the not too distant future, marriage, house purchase, stressful job, career and then middle age and it is then that lots of people wake up to the realisation that they are in trouble and that the spine needs sorting out! It is then –if the person consults an FMM practitioner—that the extent of error will be pointed out as well as the presence of a system so wonderful that it can sort out most of the problems!!! Many of these patients are angry that no-one has pointed out these features to them.
If there is a failure to deal with the pains and aches, as is the case with so many ----we estimate that one in twenty will genuinely deal with the causes and make changes to correct the errors----then adaptation will continue and old age will manifest in the manner all Westerners are accustomed to. There will be loss of height, loss of motivation and

mobility and a walking stick will become necessary. Old age will be upon the person and hip joint replacements will become an issue or a new knee will be ordered. And all this has come about without the consent of the owner and without his or her knowledge —and this is because we live surrounded by ignorance. There is greatest ignorance in the NHS, followed by the alternative health field especially amongst osteopaths and chiropractors. If this group of health care practitioners had received training in yoga at the outset then there *could* be much greater level of realisation in the populace outside of the NHS.Instead, in some osteopathic institutions it is normal to recommend avoiding yoga— especially yoga!

If we were to examine why this ignorance exists within the NHS, it is so because at all levels there is only a focus upon symptoms and their removal. There is at no time any serious attempt to search for a cause. It is irrelevant what part of the NHS one looks at -there is only absolute concentration upon symptom removal. There is nothing wrong with this and this is not intended as a criticism —but the patients are not sufficiently knowledgeable nor intelligent in the main, to be able to ask the critical question before any treatment is begun—"will what you are proposing deal with the **primary** cause of my problem??" It is a very simple question and I am sure that all honest doctors will give an equally simple answer NO to the question. But the patient does not ask, indeed is discouraged from asking anything pertinent to the cause. Now this in no way implies that there is anything inadequate about the level of care that the patent receives when treatment is underway—so many of my patients have complimented their hospital doctors for the care given as well as the nursing care. But that is not the issue we are dealing with now. No-one will be interested in WHY the patient has come to this point except in so far as such things as excess alcohol or tobacco usage will probably be spelled out. The heart attack victim will not have any understanding that posture may well have had a dramatic effect upon the heart function. No-one with asthma will be taught to perform yoga breathing by anyone in a GP surgery. The constipation sufferer will not be advised about posture, exercise, diet and so on. Of course it goes without having to be said that none of these sufferers from all the ills including bad backs and stiff necks, will be advised to take up yoga the one thing that would almost guarantee a successful outcome. The common scenario is for the patient to be offered a pill of some sort which, itself, will be stated to have significant side-effects and, if the question were asked —"will this pill remove the cause" would again elicit a NO.

Let us take a very common and simple case. Mr A is 45 years of age and underwent a knee cartilage removal at the age of 30. He does not know how much was removed nor does he understand how it is that he is able to continue without one. On presenting for treatment for spinal trouble he reports that he used to suffer frequent back and knee pain for many years and nothing was done and no-one was able to diagnose a fault. He claims to have several arthroscopies after which no abnormality was detected. Our assessment on manual examination showed extensive contracture of the hamstrings and heavily contractured calf muscles both of which have a considerable influence upon how the knee functions. No-one advised him of this despite regular visits to doctors and physios to find relief, which never came. This BASIC bit of knowledge is at the level of what we refer to as Noddys Guide!!! It is so plain and so simple yet is universally ignored—but had this man been told that short hamstrings could lead to knee trouble and that daily stretching would likely prevent this then surely many would take this up?? Perhaps we are truly naïve!!

This then, is the human condition in purely physical terms. The mental condition will also strike most people simply by the act of living in a culture almost devoid of fun and laughter. There is a level of seriousness about people that is unhealthy. The suicide rate has never been higher. There is now so much anxiety about everything from mugging, rape, bird flu, immigrants and terrorism that the whole culture seems wrapped in gloom. There seems to be little ability to rationalise the risks of each of the threats. The mental disorders and aberrations to which people subject themselves are accepted as if they were inevitable, largely mirroring the physical condition—"well, what can you do-- when you get old these things happen?" So I summarise the human condition as being that set of physical, mental and spiritual characteristics that the individual ACQUIRES and CREATES in her lifetime which could be avoided or substantially reduced and which amount to a loss of that level of health which could be expected to be maintained.

The human condition is largely that set of "troubles" which the person states are part of his life which, to the trained and experienced observer are common amongst so many other people, but that the complainer fails to see as part of life anyway. The failure to see that life just IS accounts for the greater part of the stress and anxiety of modern life despite 3000 years of philosophy and despite good housing and money in the bank and all the other benefits that modern people have that could never have been envisioned even 100 years ago. The human condition is not being able to see that life is not your troubles. Life is harmony, peace, love beauty, good fortune and all those other things that cannot be purchased nor obtained but can be created by **changes in mind-set**. Today, it is probable that the awareness of what is possible is greater than ever was the case but the vast majority do not actually pursue the ideal.

Of course, there will be those who take issue with the basic precept above—but remember that I have practised yoga for over twenty years and taught for nearly as long and have been witness to thousands of people improving their "condition" physically emotionally and spiritually, even from the most dire set of circumstances. So if you are intent upon an argument then come prepared with YOUR evidence to the contrary and be prepared to have it picked over much as a vulture would pick over the dead carcass!!

2. *Myofascial Contracture.*

Every muscle is covered in fascia. Muscles derive their directional stability from the fascia. Each set of muscle fibres is wrapped around with this material. If we take the longest muscle in the body, the quadriceps, we can find that each individual muscle belly named as vastus—lateralis, medialis and intermedius -has been wrapped with fascia. The fascial coverings are what make up the tendon which is then attached to the periosteum covering the bone. Fascia is classified as superficial and deep. The deep fascia surrounds the bones and deep muscles and the superficial is as its name implies under the skin. It is the same fascial envelope which surrounds the skull as surrounds the feet—therefore everything is connected fascially.

Fascia is a vast and complex system embedded in which is masses of blood vessels, lymph channels and nerve endings. There are many pain receptors whereas it is possible to push a needle through the actual muscle fibres without feeling much pain, these being greatly less innervated. The mechanical behaviour of fascia can be likened to a plastic carrier bag. If you take hold of the bag in both hands and take out all the slack it then becomes taught. Apply moderate force to stretch it and you will feel the elasticity. If you then remove the pulling force the material springs back to its original size. If you then apply much more pulling force there will eventually be an actual lengthening of the material—this is plastic deformation and is subject to Hooke's Law just as are all elastic materials. Steel behaves in the same way. There are thus three phases in the actual stretch process—1—take out the slack, 2—apply force to elastically deform and 3—much more force to plastically deform and actually lengthen the material. Without this third phase there is no actual stretching which is retained. Now it is vital to your learning that you understand this—that *fascia adapts itself in length to the habitual range of use to which the muscle is put*

This means that if you do not actively lengthen each muscle each day it will gradually lose its length. Now on this issue there is GENERAL CONFUSION. I put it in capitals because the response of most of my patients to this statement is---"But all this exercise I do surely it would keep me flexible". With a little thought it can be seen that this cannot be the case because exercise only repeats an already well established pattern and in fact is responsible for much of what goes wrong with fascia. Stretching takes TIME---- exercise is done QUICKLY!!! If you wish much more knowledge of fascia then you will find it in my first book "Message in the Body|"

The process of myofascial contracture is responsible for almost all the postural distortions that humans go through. There is one golden rule which is elaborated upon later in the book which essentially justifies this statement. The process of contracture is what I am concerned with here. Let us look at that which I claim is the first obvious sign in the 5 year old—hamstring shortening. When the 5 year old was one year old you could take the child and lay it down on its back and then take one leg held straight and flex it at the hip taking it to the point at which the knee touched or nearly touched the chin. This is the full **design length** of the hamstrings. Now this is not the case for all babies as some are more flexible than others which is probably genetic—but the difference is not massive. Now the 5 year old has lost around 25% of the range if we measure the range as from the knee touching the chin to the leg being laid down on the floor as it was before commencing. It could be more than 25% but unless you had checked the one year old you are not able to make that assertion. Check both legs on the 5 year old and observe that she is likely to stop you proceeding any further because it is already beginning to hurt!! The pain of stretching tissue in the human is the same for the 5 year old as for the 50 year old—probably the 50 year old is better able to cope with it because of experience whilst the 5 year old is likely to have not experienced any significant pain. In any event you can be assured that she would not allow you to stretch her hamstrings because it is too painful. The average young lad who has appeared in our clinics and in the workshops for students of fmm, if he is involved in strong sports—ours usually are—will have lost over 75% of hamstring length as measured on this scale. Observing the boy performing a forward bend will usually result in it being obvious that he is not able to touch his knees let alone his feet! Calves will be not as bad but will also need attending to

The hamstrings have shortened and the myofascial matrix surrounding the muscle bellies has adapted to the habitually used short range. This means that the muscle is behaving just as your bicep behaves if you care to observe it, during elbow flexion. You will see that as you flex your elbow to bring your hand to your shoulder; your bicep gets shorter but fatter. All muscles behave like this—so the hamstrings on the five year old have also shortened and *fattened*. Now muscle that has contracted to make a joint move is supposed to return to the relaxed position and be lengthened after the work is done—watch your bicep after you have contracted it—what do you do? –you allow your arm to relax and the arm STRAIGHTENS. It is the act of straightening that again lengthens the bicep and brings the myofascial matrix to its correct resting length. This you do automatically on your arm—but how to do it with the hamstrings? Only the forward bend will do it-so how many times a day do you perform the forward bend?? Never –is that correct? How many times a day does the 5 year old perform the forward bend? The answer is also probably not at all—but the baby probably does many times as it is learning to walk but then gives it up—but of course the baby for the first few years of life is seldom sitting on a chair; the floor is the normal place—so the hamstrings are subjected to some degree of lengthening as a result. The baby also daily performs many flexing exercises naturally. This I refer to as the innate intelligence and this characteristic is explained much more in Message in the Body and the Shanti Yoga School students manuals. The innate intelligence is what causes the cat and dog to create good health for much longer than the average human can do—but the average human has had a brilliant teacher in the form of the child but has not observed the value of the lessons! The adult prefers to acquire what is today called " training" –this formula learning is what is taught to physiotherapists and osteopaths and chiropractors which probably accounts for the low cure rate amongst their patients and the continual complaint that I receive from patients who are angry that they spent a lot of money with these therapists and got nowhere! Formula learning is that body of knowledge which is what I refer to as Internet Knowledge, the mixture of snippets of data taken from numerous sources most of whose authors of which are confused about the reason for the human body going wrong and who confuse facts with understanding. There are many examples of Internet Knowledge—we could take as a flavour of the month the issue of cholesterol which has become the new bogey man despite their being a large body of evidence that the highest cholesterol levels exist in Eastern Europeans who have the lowest rate of heart disease!! We could take another current phenomenon—the issue of dehydration. All of a sudden everyone seems to think they are dehydrated—so many yoga students are now equipped with water bottles –presumably to enable them to avoid becoming dehydrated. But let us consider the rationale. Do desert tribesmen continually drink from bottles of water? Do read Laurens van der Post –his books about the Khalahari desert dwellers should at least point you to the possibility that all this current round of thinking is another thing to be fearful about!! To become dehydrated in normal UK conditions would require a serious loss of fluid from excess exercise, for example, or simply not drinking for at least a couple of days. How arrogant it is to assume that the incredible human body is not sufficiently intelligent to let you know you need to drink by causing that old favourite –THIRST. Do you carry food around with you as well? Are you in danger of starving? Of course not—why?—because you will feel HUNGRY and this will lead you to eat!! Trust the vastly intelligent body to let you know when to DRINK as well. But many articles in magazines are written by so –called experts on such subjects. The magazine market is a hungry machine and needs feeding—its voracious appetite for "stuff" is insatiable---how else is the owner to keep himself in new BMW's? So—always we are being called, especially in today's world as never before, to CONSIDER WELL before allowing oneself to be persuaded by others.

Just as an aside, the latest round of refutations comes from an intelligent source and the subject is----low fat milk. There is now powerful evidence that low fat dieting is responsible for ovarian cancers and does not allow proper weight balancing to occur. All this is entirely contrary to what has been publicised over the past few years! It is also powerful persuasion to take certain prescription drugs.

Yoga cannot be understood by any means other than by doing it. Even then doing it does not guarantee understanding since it is only when the practitioner of yoga comes truly to let go of existing " knowledge" and allow himself to be filled with the *gnosis*, that TRUE knowledge which does not come from formal training courses. Indeed, gnosis comes only from within the individual AS A RESULT OF THE APPLICATION OF THE PRINCIPLES OF THE SYSTEM. I placed this last part in capital letters because it is still common for a patient to demand of me how I think yoga is going to help her condition when no exercise has yet done so—to which the answer is that one must DO IT to find out—but, of course, this is just not the Western way of seeing things. The Western mind wants PROOF first then and only then will action be commenced—of course this applies to those other than the dedicated small minority who somehow understand this principle without proof!

We return to the notion of myfascial contracture. The word contracture means –and it is well understood in hospitals so is not my terminology ----the permanent state of contraction of the muscle. But it seems that no-one involved in general medicine has expressed any interest in precisely what happens in this state so the term contracture is glibly used without any real appreciation of the implications and certainly not the causes.

We can take our teenage boy—boys are much worse than girls in the postural compromise stakes for reasons which I do not understand (could it be self-esteem?) and observe that each would not be able to perform a cobra posture to the same extent that was possible at the age of 5 or even 9. What would be visible would be the loss of spinal mobility at around the upper part of the spine, demonstrating the myofascial contracture at the point where the most slumping is present—so the boys are round shouldered and the clavicles are sunken, causing the head to be pushed forward and creating immobility in the lowest two vertebrae of the neck. This also must cause the lower lumbar erector spinae to become tense when they would otherwise be relaxed. They would normally be relaxed and alternately tightening and relaxing during walking but this will not happen when the head is forward simply because of the natural implications of gravity and functional characteristics. Thus, erector spinae are bound to contracture as well if the person does not lengthen them daily by performing the forward bend.

The process of myofascial contracture is happening at all the major points of great physical stress in the average human. The canoeist will have a huge degree of contracture in the trapezius after 10 years of paddling a boat. The oarsman and woman will have great contracture in the erector spinae around the mid-spine area. The serious hockey player, if he plays on Astroturf may well be suffering from restricted range in the hip joints. This is especially so if the Astroturf is laid without cushioning as was the case with many clubs—to save money!! I saw a few young men with all the signs of hip joint deterioration, in their early twenties!!—as a result of hockey on uncushioned man-made surfaces. Do bear in mind that ordinary grass has great softness and thus considerable shock absorbing capability. Also much hockey was played on grass up until very recently.

The most common sites for contracture are –and this can be considered to be a sort of league table!!-------
1. trapezius
2. erector spinae
3. pectorals
4. external/internal oblique—the corset
5. hamstrings
6. calves and tibials

Of course, included in the trapezius is the neck muscles which are affected in so many people. What one rarely sees is gluteus maximus contracture and quadriceps contracture. Also rare is forearm flexors and extensors in a state of contracture. But rare means exactly that-it does not mean that it does not occur since we have treated sufferers with these characteristics-- but statistically it is a small portion of the total.

Myofascial contracture has numerous ramifications for the whole process of human function but this subject is well covered in my other works so I suggest you refer to these. It should be sufficient to say to anyone who is awake that the effect on the whole organism is so slow and gradual that most are unaware until treatment removes the contracture. Since the average patient is back to normal within about 4or 5 session over even less weeks, you can imagine that the patient has quite a job to reconcile these changes when the whole process of contracture has taken many decades. So the evidence of the severity of the ramifications for contracture is not in the patients acquisition of the contracture which is too slow to notice but in his shedding of its effects which is dramatically rapid!! Many patients, thus, make remarks about feeling lighter or distorted or much more upright- reflections of a sudden change in "posture" for want of a better word.

3. Loss of Mobility

Once again we take the example of the baby for our point of reference. If you were to examine the spinal mobility of the baby it would be much the same as the 5 year old. You would perceive a softness of movement when attempting to move each vertebrae. If you take the arm and leg and check the movement in each of the major joints the same sort of feeling would come through your hands. You would not need to have any previous experience to feel this characteristic. If you now go through the same process with a teenager you would find muscles tougher to feel and if you watched the forward bend you would most probably see massive shortening in the hamstrings at the back of the leg. Feeling these you would immediately notice how much harder are the hamstrings than those of the 5 year old. But test the knee flexion—ask the teenager to sit on her heels on the floor and there is no difficulty—indicating that the knee is so far unaffected by this shorting process. Then ask the teenager—especially a boy –to sit between his feet and then to lie back between his feet so that his head is resting on the floor. It is likely that he will complain that the quadriceps hurt very badly as they are being strongly stretched. You might also notice that he is unwilling to actually move into this position at all or at least comes out of it very quickly declaring that it is too painful. Now sitting on the heels has shown unequivocally that the knee joints are not at all restricted but if the quads are allowed to remain tight and the hamstrings are not lengthened then there will be gradual adaptation to this situation and the knee will gradually malfunction. How this manifests is impossible to say but one of the first things to be spotted amongst those over 50 who come for treatment is their inability to flex the knee fully. This indicates that the capsule has shrunk along with the tough covering of the capsule, both being richly endowed with nerves and blood vessels. This is probably one of the most frequent sources of pain.

The justification for the major joints malfunctioning can be made entirely on the basis of the extent and frequency of full mobilisation—or the lack of it. The rather corny expression "if you don't use it you lose it" is on everyone's lips but so few of those stating this understand how it applies to themselves. Of course, it is quite easy to spot the elbow joint and the knee joint and the shoulder joint and the wrist joint beginning to lose range but the hip should let you know as soon as possible but does not do so. Consider that the hip for most modern people is subjected to no more than a 90degree mobilisation, enforced by the change from sitting to standing. On checking, many hip joints will be found to be lacking in flexion even though no symptoms appear. Many patients who perceive this loss do nothing until the appearance of pain which they take to be a serious warning!! How is it that the perceived loss of movement did not trigger action to redress the balance, before pain arrived? Well, this we may label as part of the human condition, added to a touch of the martyr in all of us. Lots of people simply soldier on, as they call it, without wanting to bother anyone!! The other explanation is that our culture—indeed Western culture generally, is full with those manifesting difficulties in movement and it is thus so common as to be hardly noteworthy. Hospitals, doctors, physios and all manner of alternative practitioners do little to help—of course, this is once again an observation of the lack of yogic understanding. Rounding up on the subject of hip joints it may be of great interest to a few to know that there are no hip joint replacements on the Indian sub-continent and two Indian surgeons that I have met confirm that this is because people sit in the cross-legged position from childhood! They also squat. This brings almost the full range of movement into play regularly, just as happens with elbow and shoulder

The understanding that there has been a loss of mobility in a hip joint, for example, is not difficult to see nor to comprehend. But the frequency of such occurrences pales when compared with that which goes wrong in so many spines—the spinal vertebrae lose movement, the process beginning at the age of around 9. Why? The reason is so simple –you have failed to keep it moving through its full range. On hearing this so many patients squeal that they have done a life time of exercises provided by physios or osteopaths so how can there be loss of movement!! There is inherent in this complaint, the superficial understanding of body function. Exercise is seen as a good thing for every problem but let us just consider one joint and see how exercise helps it. The hip joint is stiff because it has not been used throughout its entire range—the range has not been used so it has been lost, so to speak. What exercise would fully flex the hip joint??? What exercise would satisfy the yogic criteria of holding the position while the myofascial structures actually length---this is what I call a proper stretch ---which takes at least 30 secs?? Naturally there is not one system of exercise that can do this—so the person demonstrates his ignorance largely fuelled by those who call themselves exercise professionals who are also ignorant and who have been taught by those who also do not know!! This is how the ignorance has been perpetuated—but there is a feature of all this that is far more worrying—there are so few, regardless of how many degrees they have or years of medical training, that are capable of asking the most important question –how is what you have proposed for exercise going to make my joints less stiff? To be able to ask such a searching question of a physio or osteopath or chiropractor would imply that the patient knew something about the condition with which she is afflicted—hereby lies the problem—the patients are as ignorant as the practitioners and are readily willing to listen and act upon the most dubious of instructions. I have seen sets of instruction from professionals that are a real indication that the patient has had the Mickey taken out of them—some have been asked to perform the most ludicrous of movements which, it goes without saying, have produced no effect. Now to give someone exercises which the practitioner knows full well are a joke seems to be inconceivable, leaving no other logical conclusion than ignorance of the condition of the patient and thus, ignorance of what will work to rectify it is the true picture. I prefer to believe in the sincerity of purpose of health professionals rather than believe in the notion of deliberate deceit. Therefore, ignorance is the only logical explanation.

Now we come to that which causes 97% of the trouble. The spine. The spine is the master system, the legs and arms are the slaves. There are no organs or systems in the limbs so everything that happens in one of them must be the result of some central disturbance—which means the spine. This is what the yogis understood thousands of years ago—hence yoga postures are entirely aimed at working the spine and the abdominal contents—the source of all disease and dysfunction. Aside, naturally, from those accidents and diseases which could focus on limbs --these are rare. Here we refer to the average patient or pain sufferer. How does the spine lose its mobility??—in just the same way as the hip joint, but the signs for the patient are critically few. You should consider that the spine in its horizontal form is perfect for its purpose. In the horizontal position, all the forces are equal along the entire length and each abdominal organ hangs from it just as clothes in a wardrobe. But tip the" wardrobe" through 90degrees and the effect is disastrous for the owner. Now this matters very little if you happen to be a tribesman living in the Amazon jungle because you will be living an entirely natural life with lots of resting and lots of hunting which involves long periods spent running after game. This natural life reduces the prospect of what are referred to as the diseases of civilisation—heart disease, diabetes, arterial hardening, muscle wasting, constipation—the list is endless. And this natural life reduces the risk of any spinal trouble just because of this naturalness. But sit this same warrior in front of a computer, in a car, give him a few years of stress and appalling diet and you would see precisely the same disorders of the spine. Indeed, this phenomenon has been observed on the Indian subcontinent by Western trained doctors who proclaim that the diseases of the Westerner soon become normal for the Indian who chooses to live as the Westerner, adopting a Western –style diet and way of life— including the use of chairs to sit on!! (Just this week a BBC broadcast programme heralded the huge explosion in diabetes in Indians who are becoming obese, the narrator placing the blame immediately and squarely on poor diet and lack of exercise.)

This enables the principle to be expressed—unless there is constant mobilisation of joints there will be hardening and shrinkage of the structure around each joint wherever it lies. If there is inadequate mobilisation of the abdominal organs there will be adhesions and poor blood flow leading to pathological changes. This is the root of all ailments aside from that real killer—the mind!! But we shall come to that.

4. The Congestive Condition

What actually happens when a joint loses some of its range of movement? The simplest way to see what is happening is to picture joints just like any other flow system—there has to be material coming in and material being transported out. What is coming in to the joint is replacement materials for those used up—repairs and maintenance if you prefer. All living structure act like this—but it is no different from what happens to you, the owner of the body. Each day you go to the toilet and get rid of that which is not needed—recognise that half of the material waste is dead skin cells!--- but it is vital that you eat in order to replenish that which has been lost and consumed. So the nutrients in the food provide the repair material for the body to be maintained properly. Now each joint requires its share of this nutrient—how is it to receive it if there is no movement between the surfaces around the joint? Movement is the prime stimulus just as muscle contraction is the prime stimulus for blood to flow around the whole pipework system. Each spinal vertebra has around itself, lots of fascia and little short muscles and ligaments binding it to its fellows above and below. Each of these structures requires movement to fully function. With this arrangement it can be concluded that all these elements require lengthening –they need stretching as this is the action that helps to maintain the movement of repair materials—as well as shortening. This is a constant ebb and flow. When there is inadequate movement and stiffness and associated pain, we have what we refer to as congestion. The evidence for the presence of such a phenomenon is when we mobilise the joint, the pain immediately reduces and as soon as there is full mobility there is no pain—this is the common scenario. Of course, the vertebra and its adjoining structures, are not counted as joints because they do not have synovia and thus do not produce fluid for lubrication. The apophyseal joints, the facets, **are** synovial joints so there is a distinct possibility of these, which are part of each vertebrae, to become strained just like a knee or hip joint. We must also not forget that each rib is attached at two joints either side of each of the 12 thoracic vertebrae—and these are also synovial joints.

But there is another much more invasive and insidious disaster waiting to happen—it is the intervertebral disc which does not receive sufficient movement unless yoga is performed. It is immediately debatable whether this feature of the spine should warrant a special section all on its own simply because of the seriousness with which it should be considered.

The ignorance of the need to constantly mobilise the IVD 's (intervertebral discs) by compression and decompression alternately, is universal. The fact that the disc deteriorates is well known amongst all professional physical therapists --- but it can seem an entirely theoretical bit of knowledge. If this was not the case every doctor and physio and osteopath and chiropractor—and all other physical therapists would surely give all their patients the discipline of yoga to perform. They would have explained the mechanism of disc deterioration which would automatically lead the recipient to conclude that he had best do something about this for the future. But there is no professional body which is known to recommend yoga, it being the only process which will satisfy the body!! Indeed of all the many people I have treated who had serious disc problems and have had physical therapy in many forms, no one person has ever understood the mechanism of disc degeneration. Not even the surgeons after performing spinal surgery inform the patient as to what has gone wrong.

Let us examine what is the mechanism of disc degeneration. It is straightforward---- the disc is considered to be inert. Which means that there is no "life" in it in the same way that there is life in a joint or other cellular parts. The disc is filled with fluid and has its construction identical to a modern radial ply tyre on a car. In fact, the Michelin X tyre of the past, which was tested on the Paris metro trains, was modelled on the construction of the human disc because of its **inherent strength.**

We are not talking of a weak structure, as witnessed by the fact that the circus strongman can hold six other humans on his shoulders without the disc bursting. The human disc when it is in good condition—this is medically tested --is capable of withstanding over 1000lb. of weight per square inch. Six men on your shoulders must amount to at least 60 stone—this is over 800 pounds weight. It should help to dispel the modern myth about people being weak or the body being incapable of managing heavy loads. Now we can consider what happens to the disc--- let us start with lying down. You are in bed. Your spinal discs automatically fill up with new fluid drawn from the bone either side, diffusing through the end-plate of each vertebra. This, of course will only happen if the vertebra is mobile. This is akin to pumping up the car tyre. This explains why each person is taller on rising—the discs are more hydrated. You rise from your nights sleep and immediately the discs begin to empty their watery content, into the waste disposal system, again using the bony end plate. The old material is gradually squeezed out during the day and again replenished at night. The whole process is known as **nocturnal imbibition—night time drinking!**

What medical researchers have found is that if the disc is kept compressed or decompressed, there is deterioration of the structure, what can be classified on an MRI scan as degeneration. What has not been understood is WHY this occurs—we believe that there is overwhelming evidence that the effect occurs because the individual has failed to keep the vertebrae sufficiently mobile. This may also explain why it occurs so frequently at L5/S1 and L5/L4—this is the place of maximum compression and L5 commonly seizes up. If L5 seizes up –it becomes completely immobile—it follows that its position is one of compression – that is, it is nearer to the sacrum than would be the case if it were free to move. Lying down at night, the spine is preparing for all discs to refill with new fluid but L5 will have this nocturnal imbibition interfered with simply because it is not able to permit the disc to expand. And that is because all the little muscles and ligaments have shortened thus holding the vertebra closer to the sacrum even though the compression has been removed.

Not only will the disc gradually degenerate but there will also be a congestion around all the little structures which form part of the articulation. And it is this which may also produce symptoms which could just as easily be explained by disc deterioration. This may require explanation. The congestive condition can be likened to a building site at which many lorries deliver bricks—and, of course, bricklayers are laying them. This is a flow system-all human endeavour has the same principles. But what would happen if the brick layers all decided to stop work— assuming the lorries continued to arrive because this is what is already programmed (the equivalent is for repair materials to be continually sent to the site in the body) –it is almost certain that congestion would occur. The pallets of bricks would soon pervade the whole site and it would become clogged up—congestion!! Whilst the human body systems are vastly more complex than work systems the principals remain valuable if you are to understand the mechanism of congestion. Damming up a river is another example. These concepts are accepted within the field of physical medicine but it is certain that no-one has specific knowledge that this is actually what happens simply because no tests have been done on living subjects only on cadavers. Old osteopathic text books make the same claim although without the justification.

Let us return to our disc—it is the presence of gradually deteriorating mobility which starts to interfere with nocturnal imbibition and once the compression/ decompression axis is compromised deterioration is inevitable. But we have to say that this is conjecture and not irrefutable fact. The nature of this degeneration is often referred to, by radiologists and medics alike, as "wear and tear". This epithet is perhaps appropriate to man-made machinery—or perhaps the car tyre. But wear and tear is a distinct function of use whereas degeneration in the human spine, when it is not universal but local, must be the result of **too little** movement rather than an excess. As for the tear, whilst it is endemic to human tissue that tearing takes place, around the tendonous attachments in certain areas, this does not contribute to degeneration. The fact of degeneration, selective as it usually is, can be traced almost entirely to the interference to normal function of the nocturnal imbibition phenomenon. This results in the addition of congestion and possibly irritation of nerves. It may be this irritation that creates the natural splint so common in humans. This is the inflammatory response—there may be a slight tear in a piece of fascia or one of the little rotator muscles around a joint or it could possibly be on the more gross level and be located in erector spinae muscles, for example The inflammation causes splinting of the local area to prevent the person from causing further trouble. Then this turns into an increase in immobility which becomes permanent, simply because the owner has failed to perceive the loss of movement. This immobility creates congestion and there is the beginning of spinal disc degeneration by virtue of an interference in the suck/squeeze effect from consistent daily compression followed by decompression. Since this is the sole route for new nutrients to reach the disc—there are no blood vessels nor any nerves in the disc—it follows that degeneration must take place. But this must be seen as it really is –this is not wear and tear which does not feature in the human body. Parts do not wear away in normal use otherwise the first victim would be the joints of the feet—these suffer very little degeneration whilst the spine is the principal victim of deterioration in all forms. This may give some food for thought to those convinced that arthritis-or the degenerative condition labelled as such but which should more properly have the title arthrosis-is the result of overuse. It is not—if anything it results from underuse since it is mostly a disorder inherent to Westerners whose diet is execrable, usually—so maybe the evidence of foot bones not suffering much from arthrosis could help some to realise the truth of arthritis and arthrosis.

We will add some highly technical detail about the human disc. The central part of the disc is termed the nucleus pulposus. It is gelatinous, being 88% water which is strongly hydrophilic and chemically made up of a mucopolysaccaride matrix. The nucleus is composed of collagenous fibres and is tightly bounded by fibrous tracts termed the annulus fibrosus. These are made up of concentric fibres which appear to cross one another obliquely. The central fibres in contact with the nucleus are nearly horizontal running between the vertebral plateux in ellipsoidal fashion. The nucleus is thus contained by a series of inextensible fibres.

The notion held within the medical scientific world is that in the young this is so well integrated that prolapse is impossible but I have witnessed two L5/S1 disc ruptures on rowers not yet 21.

The nucleus is held under pressure even when unloaded so that if the disc is cut with a knife the pulp becomes extruded even though there is no load. This probably makes it mechanically more efficient at load distribution. There is more to be said about the water in the disc since this part will help greatly to demonstrate the extent to which modern science has ignored reality and this reality is known and has been known by science for many decades. This part demonstrates this.

The nucleus rests on the vertebral plateau an area lined by cartilage which is full of microscopic pores linking the casing of the nucleus and the spongy bone underlying the vertebral plateau. When a significant force is applied to the spinal column, as during standing, the water contained with the gelatinous matrix of the nucleus escapes into the vertebral body through these pores. As this static pressure is maintained throughout the day, by night the disc is perceptibly thinner and in a normal healthy person this can have created 2cm loss of overall height. Conversely, during the night, whilst lying flat there is an exponentially rapid change in height –in other words it is a rapid increase in thickness which slows down with time. If the forces of applied load and removed load are made too quickly the disc is considered to not attain its proper resting thickness and this state is considered to be *analogous to ageing.*

We consider this is the state to which many people subject themselves unwittingly –too much sitting, with too little relief from sitting. So far concentration has been upon the notion of joint congestion, which I feel is relatively easy to understand. What may not be quite so simple to follow is how muscles come to have the same label applied—bearing in mind that it is I applying such a label. Here is a common example that will be recognised by all students and practitioners of fmm, from the earliest days of training. The almost-vertical fibres of the trapezius which attach to the lowest vertebrae of the thoracic spine and which overlap the latisimus dorsi at this level, overlay the erector spinae fibres which run north to south right up against the spine. A little higher at around the southern border of the scapula, the rhomboids are attached to the spine and to the scapula and draw the scapula towards the spine. At around this same level is the serratus posterior muscle. Let us take all four of these and see that each has its own function. This function must be independent of the surrounding muscles even though there is co-dependence. No muscle functions in isolation. Now it is the fmm therapist who can testify to the presence, in many patients, of virtual immobility of this area of the body. Palpating that area between the vertebral border of the scapula—the lower part of it—and the spine, it is possible to deduce from the feel of the tissue, that there is what we describe as glueing together of all the structures. This can be felt as a substantial mass which is also attached to the underlying ribs. The whole mass cannot be moved and therapists often state to the patient that it feels like concrete!! Gradually with treatment which is deep within the tissue, this glueing can be broken down so that the muscles feel normal. This you may say is not very helpful to the yoga teacher nor to the student because they are not therapists. This we cannot counter as a criticism except to advise that sometimes this can be observed in the person who has great difficulty in performing certain posture. We will, of course, elaborate upon this later. At this juncture we want to let you know that these characteristics exist-with this in mind we set out a few more common areas for heavy congestion of myofascial structures. That which has already been outlined is indeed the most common. Probably the next most common form is at the supraspinatus which sits atop the scapula. This muscle starts the arm abduction after which the deltoid takes over. But it underlies the trapezius, this time the horizontal fibres. The average therapist will recognise that few people have no problem at this part largely because of sitting and typing or driving or using any desk bound machine. The muscle is in continuous use but is held in constant tension rather than used as muscle was designed for—to tighten and relax. Which neatly leads to the primary reason for contracture—shortening but not being lengthened sufficiently.

So our trapezius and underlying supraspinatus are almost bound to contracture in anyone sitting and using their arms outstretched without actually making the muscles work hard. The imposition of weight upon this already flawed position makes the problem much worse even thought the muscles are being made to work. The weight training makes them work too hard and then gives them no respite, no lengthening nor any proper relaxation. But this is another issue!!

Next on the list of priorities, on the basis of frequency, is probably the pectoralis major muscle which drags the head forward and glues the ribs together at the sternal position. —and probably causes the head and neck and the clavicles to malfunction. Then we move to gluteals and then to TFL or iliotibial band. This is very interesting as a problem since it causes havoc with knees! The TFL can be palpated along the lateral edge of the femur and often it has so much contracture that it has glued itself to the femur and to the hamstrings along their lateral edge. The TFL is rather like an orchestra conductor—the whole limb is dependent upon this muscle to work properly—which really means that it must be soft and relaxed and certainly not adherent to the underlying structures. If there is adherence in this way the femur will be disturbed and its function altered. This will then cause the knee to run "out of true". This is a frequent problem with runners amongst whom there is great ignorance. The TFL has only a small muscle, the band being almost solely fascia—it is a tendon. The small muscle actuating it is on the pelvis just forward of the gluteus maximus and is seen to be part of this muscle.

In the pecking order, we can now come to the gastrocnemius and its underlying soleus for which characteristics similar to those already outlined are pertinent. This feature of these two muscles often causes foot symptoms. The two muscles can be viewed as the engine of the foot and rather as the TFL is the conductor of the thigh, so the calf muscles are the conductor of the complex unit, the foot.

These observation are of course, purely from the perspective of the therapist and it is the fact that we are therapists as well as being yoga teachers that has enabled us to bring this level of detail to bear upon our work in yoga. We would be ready to submit that this level of knowledge could not have come about just using yoga.

Which brings us conveniently to the next facet of morbidity.

5. Irritation/Inflammation

If the concept of congestion meets with approval then we need to examine how pain is produced. Pain is the only means of recognising that there is something wrong. It would be perfectly logical to opine that anyone could surely recognise a gradually deteriorating posture, for example? But no-one has ever consulted me about loss of postural quality. Surely someone would recognise that their body had become much stiffer—but no-one has ever offered this as a reason for coming to see me as a therapist—nor indeed have yoga students come to solve such problems.. It is ONLY PAIN that brings people despite the many who do come saying that they had recognised loss of posture or less mobility – or whatever it was. But it is only the onset of pain that brings them. Tracing patterns of pain from the past, whilst listening to the patients' history, generally reveals that warnings have been given many times and they have been ignored. The statement that is common is that "after a couple of days of pain, it went away—so I thought it had repaired itself. " Of course, the practitioner has the experience to ask the obvious question----what was it then? If this is asked, inevitably the answer is "I don't know!" Often I put forward a comparable scenario-suppose you hear a rattle in your car—do you, even as it gets worse, leave it until something falls off? What do you do if the noise eventually goes away-would you trust your car on a long trip? Would you have it investigated? Few people shrug their shoulders and say they would not be bothered if the car did something similar to that done by their body. The great majority would sort out the problem—but fail to do so with body problems—UNLESS AND UNTIL they do not go away. Sleep deprivation is almost a guarantee that the person will then, at last, try to find a solution.

So—may be all these signs have been coming for a long time but have been dismissed rather than ignored. Many patients claim that they learn to live with a certain level of pain or immobility. This is especially the case as people come past middle age—wherever that point is on each persons graph. This process often engages the complicity of medical staff who simply issue pain killers seldom with any desire to understand the origin of the pain. The issuing of pain killers is often itself accompanied by the suggestion that age is a factor!

Irritation within the context of a spinal articulation is hard to define in words and this difficulty is matched by one in trying to show the presence of such a characteristic to the patient. But there are general guidelines that emerge from the therapeutic situation. Suppose the patient has nothing more than an L5 seizure—this can be easily felt by a therapist even in the first year of training. On pressing the vertebra during the assessment the person complains of pain as a result of pressure from the palpating finger or thumb. If the practitioner repeats the pressure on the vertebra and then moves to those other vertebrae closer to the head---moving to L4 and L3 and so on, but no pain is produced other than at L 5 then one can reasonably conclude that what exists is irritation or inflammation. Is this irritation from immobility? Or is this inflammation? How is it possible to ascertain which, if either, exists. Generally, it can be reasonably reliably achieved by the process of treatment. If on mobilising the vertebra it becomes considerably freer quite quickly—maybe even as the patient steps off the couch he says that he has already less pain and this is matched by the practitioners statement that the joint is moving – perhaps—25% better.-this could be interpreted as purely irritative. This would qualify as a congestive condition, which, because of local failure to move materials quickly to provide better local nutriment, has turned into an irritable joint. There may well be some inflammation as well although because the place of inflammation is several inches below the palpating thumb, one is left with pure conjecture. You might call this educated guess work.

If there is inflammation it is not possible to know except over a period of around 7-10 days of treatment time. Suppose the patient has been treated for this stiff joint on a Monday and returns for a further session on the following Thursday—a common pattern for me—and at this second session the joint is fully mobilised. Suppose then that the patient returns about 10 -14 day after the first session and reports a gradual lessening of the symptoms over roughly this period, I would conclude that this was an inflammatory condition and pain removal was not produced by the act of mobilising the joint but simply by relieving congestion.. If one permits the body, via good mobilising, to continue to do its proper job, it will "reward" the owner by reducing pain right away—but it will follow a pattern which is distinctly not the pattern of cure for those conditions which respond purely to mobilisation. Perhaps, since this may seem like a semantic argument—or that we are debating lots of "so what?" situations, it would be helpful to elaborate upon this phenomenon in the hope that it may aid understanding. Suppose our patient has L5 immobility and after the first session is getting 25% better movement assessed by the palpating hand, there is according to him a commensurate reduction in pain and that this is repeated linearly until the joint is fully mobile and the pain is no longer present. This would suggest that the condition was purely congestive and irritative but not inflammatory. When the patient has the signs of inflammation it can be only seen retrospectively, at the end of the treatment process, and the joint may be fully mobilised but the pain is still around but declining at its own pace. These type of situations make up about 5% of patients, not much more.

How does this help the yoga teacher with her students in class? If the student approaches the teacher and states a condition in her body, by observation it may be possible to offer an opinion as to the nature of the problem.—if pain comes and quickly subsides, then one could probably state that this is an inflammatory condition but something which has a gradual onset and seems to not be getting better nor worse is not going to be an inflammatory condition. If the student reports that the problem seems to have solved itself without recourse to any particular action, then inflammation is a reasonable assertion. If there is a sudden onset and the condition remains then the teacher could observe the student for signs and clues as to the nature of the problem and then propose solutions. Generally this means asking the student to work harder in a certain posture, watching for progress. More of this later in the book

Inflammation and irritation are most readily definable within the context of the "trapped nerve". This is a favourite amongst all who seek professional help-the notion of the trapped nerve has been espoused for a very long time. It has very little literal credibility-but it can on some people be shown to be present on an MRI scan. The favourite situation is for the MRI to show that there is a bulging disc which can be clearly seen. The radiologist has then usually in her report stated that the nerve root is being squeezed by the bulge from the disc. Even this is conjecture since the presence of a bulge and a nerve trunk underneath the disc bulge does not dictate that the nerve is being affected. The presence of limb symptoms would strengthen the case for saying that there is nerve compression but it should not allow you to be dogmatic. But let us say that a person has low back pain with immobility and foot symptoms especially down the back of the calf and into the heel, this would certainly incline the practitioner of physical therapy to state the strong likelihood of a disc bulge or herniation—classic sciatica. If the MRI shows clearly the presence of a piece of the disc pressing against the nerve trunk or nerve root then even then this should not blind the investigator to the possibility of a further cause or at least the possibility of another element in the equation. Frequently this can be spasm in the erectore spinae muscles which could well be the primary cause of all the other symptoms. To add further confusion, these symptoms which we may loosely call "sciatic" can also be produced by a hip joint problem and sacro-iliac joint immobility.

Let us conclude this part by saying that irritation and inflammation are unprovable ideas for you play with –they are real but you cannot know how real because you have only your eyes and to some extent your hands. This is not enough to know for certain if there is irritation or inflammation. Keep at the forefront the questions that help you to avoid being deflected or pushed off the scent—what will do this is Internet Knowledge.! In this context I mean to refer to that collection of facts, statistics theories etc which when put together are intended to inform the reader but which generally mislead the reader into considering that the collection of symptoms they locate matches those that their subject has— and thus they must have the right answer! The best question to ask is always—"how do you **know?**"

Let us conclude this section by saying that you are gaining understanding of how and why yoga affects people universally and brings better health and these pieces of knowledge we give should be seen as pieces of a jig – saw puzzle and not as a series of answers.

6. Stress, Poor Diet, etc

The word stress must surely be the most used word today—certainly there can be no magazine which does not deal with some aspect of stress—whether it is at work or in the home. It is also much abused—or shall we say inappropriately used. It is generally used in a negative or derogatory manner—that is it is seen as something to be avoided or certainly something to consider as entirely destructive. But what is meant by stress is, of course, neither positive nor negative. Stress is simply the application of forces to cause reaction. So if you apply stress to metal or wood there will be some reaction. If you put a wooden plank across two chairs and walk along the plank this will stress the wood—if it is strong enough to carry your weight but not so thick that no reaction is witnessed then there will be some amount of bend as you walk along it—this is stressing the wood. The same characteristic is apparent in all man made and natural materials when subjected to load, however it is applied. Stress, therefore, is neither good nor bad. Stress when applied to people is also neither good nor bad-it just is. The business executive who creates a dynamic business which is successful and gives her or him great stimulus for the creative spark, has been subjected to stress. But if you asked the person does stress "get you down" as the saying goes, the answer would be a clear no. The person would say that the business is exciting and he or she loves the buzz—but this is still stress. The employee who hates the job and is put upon to take on more work than he can manage but with the fervent hope of being noticed for promotion, suddenly finds himself having a nervous breakdown—at least that is what it would most likely be called—he has also been subjected to the same kind of stress.

Both people may well be what is often referred to as Type A personality—high achievers but one manages to deal well with the stress and the other becomes sick. Aside from the obvious fact that no two people are the same the primary difference between the two for our analytical purposes may well be that one is in charge of her stress and the other has it imposed from outside. One may well be a candidate for a heart attack and other for a long and happy life during and after the successful business is no longer part of life. Interviews with successful business executives in major international corporations reveals that few have any real difficulty with the stresses even though they are certain to be on a much grander scale than the struggling ladder –climber of our earlier example. Of course, one could easily say that the well paid exec. can afford to have the way of life that reduces the stresses and that the struggling ladder- climber lives in a one bedroom flat and has to make extensive use of credit cards just to survive. Undoubtedly low income creates extra difficulties but if one were to look purely at the obvious stressors at work then the business exec, has many times the forces working against him or her than the lowly employee. So we have to look to the way the mind works to find true analytical truths in our differently challenged people. The first thing might be to ask the struggling person— if you had plenty of money what would you do? My experience of asking this of lots of patients is –I DON'T KNOW! The next question asked is do you have a great desire to do anything else—do you have a burning desire to make something or create a new business or make sculptures or turn wood??? The answer is still no. But if you were to ask the business executive what her or she would do if money did not have to be earned, the answer would be that they would do what they are doing at present. That is to say that they enjoy what they do and if they did not they would do something else. But my experience is that it is only the burning desire that motivates and that dissatisfaction with ones current lot is never a motivator to change. It is the burning desire to do some other thing that motivates. And asking the disgruntled person who is struggling and then gets sick to state what they would do given different circumstances produces a shrug of the shoulders. They have no vision of what they would like to do-so are—or feel so—obliged to accept what is offered. Surveys that have been carried out amongst the UK population have demonstrated that few people are contented with life and with their employment. Lots of expressions of dissatisfaction centre around the urge for more money but this has been researched and this has been found to be the obvious manifestation of dissatisfaction but not the real problem. The real problem has been found to be—people don't feel they have a choice. They therefore find themselves well paid but struggling within a system that does not allow them to be themselves but makes it too attractive financially for an easy escape. We might conclude, then, that the stress is not caused by low income (although obviously for some this has to be the case alone) but by unresolvable stress. The executive can resolve the stress if she chose—she could leave and go elsewhere, at least that is what she considers is the case. Thus she does not consider the stress to be a "bad thing"—indeed this type of person considers that she thrives on the stress. So for one person stress kills and for the other stress invigorates. Surely this must be considered a feature of the human mind and not a feature of the material world since all are, these days, subjected to similar stressors.

What can be noted, from the purely musculoskeletal point of view, is that the fascia is affected more by adrenalin than by any other naturally occurring chemical in the human body. It hardens the fascia like no other activity or substance—it may well be the presence of excess adrenalin in the blood that produces the nervous breakdown, since adrenalin is the chemical that is vital for the flight and fight response, necessary if one is to escape from danger, but of little value in the work place. Daily drip-feeding with adrenalin may well be the real killer and not the stress.

Diet is another of those issues that is so prolifically written about today that it would be hard to make valuable comment. What the keen observer can deduce, however, from travelling around is that the British are fatter than ever before and so are the Americans. Obesity is now cited as the prospective number one killer of the current generation.

So what is the problem with diet. We consider that there are three basic issues. The first is that the human body is designed for movement, for action. It is very unwilling to adapt to the immobile lives that so many lead. Only in the last 50 years has there been a revolution in travel, to the point where many British people would admit to seldom going anywhere by foot or bike –always by car. The old joke about going to post a letter by car is no longer a joke but a reality—many state that they generally go by car for a simple short journey that could easily be achieved on foot or by bike. It is surely not necessary today to say that exercise is the only way that the human being has of using the food consumed in the manner intended. If one looks at the health of tribal people—and enough of these people exist for this to have been done by many researchers around the world- it is plain that high blood pressure, diabetes, atherosclerosis, arthritis---what are called the diseases of civilisation—are not in evidence in these people. Visiting Africa even though there are many AIDS sufferers and much poverty and desolation it is rare to see a fat person. All have to carry out hard manual tasks, the sort of tasks that have been done for thousands of years. This is one of the two major elements of weight control—exercise. The next is what is consumed. To examine the peasant diet, lauded as the best for good overall health, one only has to look at what is consumed and how it is acquired. This can easily be done in European countries such as Spain and Italy and France. These nations use 3-4 times as much fresh vegetables as the British. There are markets all over the country with much less supermarket domination than we have. So the market purchasing is part of the normal daily round for many Europeans. When we travel to these countries we see that the daily walk to the baker to pick up bread is part of the untutored health routine—people move much more slowly and take more time to eat meals and relax.

But there is one massively important factor not observed by all researchers, or at least not picked out as of vital importance—LIFE. The vegetables and fruit are full of LIFE. The fresh onion and raw tomato with cheese and freshly baked bread that is the staple of the Spanish worker –or was until mass employment and mass car usage---was full of life force, *vital force*. There is never any need to consider vitamin (which means vital amino) content nor mineral content, when one has acquired FRESH AND NATURAL produce because nature has bestowed on all fresh and natural produce the requisite proportions and quantities of these products. The Hippocratean dietary statement was this—"eat everything fresh whilst it still is, eat everything that rots before it does" This is the edict followed by the modern naturopath with modifications for modern people. But the value of the edict is not lost just because we have fast food and processing. In fact the need to search for the correct fresh food has never been greater—simply because there is so much interference with the "natural" that one can only go to the organic produce to find that which has not been interfered with. Even then there is no guarantee that the produce will be fresh nor that it will be full of vital aminos since much of the soil in the UK is classified as almost completely denuded of vitality and thus proper nutrient. This may well explain the modern phenomenon of queues of people waiting for allotments to become vacant. Twenty years ago there was a serious shortage of takers for allotment—now there are many more people who want them than there are units available. In fact the allotment culture was always considered as something of a joke—the allotment is where the disgruntled old fogey went to get away from his wife. This is not the case today—there are now many co-operatives operating, in which groups of keen like-minded people garden for vegetables so that they can be sure of the quality of the produce. This is certainly a reaction to the modern trend towards spraying chemicals onto all the vegetables to kill unwanted insects. Now these same insects are seen as friendly and the modern gardener does not wish to kill because she knows that the produce benefits even though it may not look as good as it does from off the supermarket shelf. What the modern knowing person has decided is that he will not allow his body to be polluted by chemicals-growing your own veg is the obvious way to dictate what happens. In the year 2000 I and a Dutch woman started a veg growing co-op and the 6 allotments produce for 12 people plenty of great tasting produce! This is still functioning today and is still an important part of our weekly routines.

The word diet is now taken to mean deprivation in some form—giving up something or making radical change to what is eaten. This is a misinterpretation of the word or a misuse. Diet is simply that which you eat—dieting is thus the act of deprivation whereas what is intended by the word is nothing more than a statement of what is consumed. The word would never have been used by Italians or French or Spaniards—because of their fundamentally healthy way of eating, retained amongst the majority still today. We have gone much more towards the American way of life and are now reaping the rewards. We see an NHS that cannot cope with the quantity of people who are ill and there will never be enough money to solve the health problems of the nation partly because the average diet is so awful. The political will needed to solve the problem cannot exist within a country in which so many are dependent upon drugs issued by doctors, car usage, soft living, lack of exercise, and hand-outs. We have acquired the American way—junk food made in mass catering establishments, food imported by persons unknown and grown in conditions unknown, lifeless soil, no real husbandry in vegetable growing, heavy mechanisation in farming –the list could go on. This is a serious health disaster for all British people –there is no wonder that the health service is groaning under the weight of bodies waiting for treatment. The absurdity of this way of life cannot, it would appear, be seen by politicians. There would appear to be no discussion about the banality of extracting huge tax revenues from the use of alcohol and tobacco to fuel the ever growing demand for disease reducing services. The irony cannot surely be lost on all politicians?

To summarise—the human condition is worsened by the use of food that has no life. Tinned, packetted, ready-prepared, frozen—all these mechanisms are a disaster for LIVING food, for VITALITY. If you visit an African country you see vigorous people everywhere—examine the people around you in the UK and see if you can find anyone over the age of 25 who appears to have vitality. Poor diet affects every cell in the body. The replacement regime inherent in the human body—replenish all the dying cells –relies heavily upon the quality of the nutrients put in. If these are heavily polluted by chemicals this will interfere with the neuroreceptors. The average supermarket carrot, recently tested by Elm Farm Research Centre, contains 57 TIMES LESS VIATMIN A than one grown organically. What does this mean?—you have to eat a lot of carrots before you have acquired enough Vitamin A for the body to be satisfied! There is now a reappearance of rickets in UK-, not seen since war time. This is a vitamin A and D deficiency –it is now reappearing in children!!! The explanation put forward by medical professionals is poor diet linked to an excess of suncream! Vitamin A and D require sunshine directly on the skin to convert the oils to vitamins but parents are so anxious about preventing sun reaching the child's skin that cream completely stops all vitamin conversion.

I can end this section condensing the essence of Dr Steve Nugent's many dissertations on the subject of glyconutrients; "Hard working intelligent people who study to become dieticians are not being taught this crucial data. Neither are doctors. They do not learn that losses of vital nutrients from foods are far greater than they could imagine. To compound the problem our foods are harvested green to improve the shelf life but only ripe fruit has the necessary quantity of nutrients.

Heart disease is the number one killer in USA and UK and the soils are depleted of selenium, just as an example. This substance is vital for heart health. The US Senate in 1936 said "The alarming fact is that foods are being grown on soils seriously depleted of nutrient. No matter how much of the food we eat it is impossible to gain enough valuable trace elements. Some foods are of no value at all"

Organic food is the best way to gain the nutrient especially if you are a meat eater. All the animals on a certified organic farm are not fed any antibiotics nor do they consume applied chemicals on the grass. This is especially important as the grass fed animals store all the chemical toxins in their liver so that eating the animal directly causes the consumer to partake of the poisons accumulated in the animal. Organically grown animals also have a much leaner meat, --the fat stores the chemical poisons. Modern factory farming methods cause the consumer to consume all the accumulated poisons which are contained within the animal. What must be recognised now is that poisons in the atmosphere cannot be avoided by anyone-therefore organic produce must of necessity contain some of the chemical poisons man has made-but the organic movement works very hard at avoiding the use of any chemicals, therefore the amounts are much smaller than in mass produced fruit and vegetables.

The next issue is that raw food is much higher in nutrient. For example, an organic carrot loses ALL its vitamin A when cooked---as well as the vitamin E and the tocopherols.

7. Poor Breathing—Diaphragmatic Compromise

Inherent in the upright position for humans, is the need for all to lift the rib cage to create an in- breath. The four legged animal does not have to do this—the ribs naturally fall open for inspiration whilst expulsion involves lifting the ribs. This itself renders the four legged animal much more efficient in the use of diaphragm breathing. Watch a cat when it is lying down—see that the breathing is all solely diaphragmatic—there is no movement in the upper part of the body, it is all visible at the stomach area. Watch the average human and you will see dominance of the clavicular breathing pattern. Ask the person to take a deep breath and watch that the upper ribs immediately lift. There is no obvious movement at the diaphragm. If you were to take the cat even in advanced old age and gently squeeze the rib cage it would be as flexible as it was in its youth—try this on a fifty year old man and prepare to be horrified! This is why the yogis of old considered it so important that proper breathing was taught. However, if you watch a child you will see the true animal state in action all the time—the child does not have to be told to breath using the diaphragm, as it always does this. There is a loss around teenage as the person becomes more immobile, more desk bound. How does this come about for the average person? The answer can be easily be found by observing the beginners in a yoga class. Observe that while attempting the camel posture, kneeling down and opening the chest, the lower parts of the ribs are close together. You can see that the width of the clavicular part of the chest is much broader than the breadth at the base of the ribs. Study, then, the child and you will quickly see that the base of the ribs is much broader than at the clavicular part. Further observation whilst both the new yogi and the child are taking a full breath, will reveal that the child has massive lower rib movement while the adult has none. What has happened?- the rectus abdominus muscles have fascially shrunk so much that they are acting as a corset around the lower ribs and having exactly the same effect as the old fashioned bodice which women wore to make their hour –glass shape. The difference, of course, is that the corset could be removed at night. The fascialy shrunk corset, formed by the fascial shortening of internal/external oblique muscles as well as the transversalis, is a gradually applied muscular tourniquet, with far more serious results than would be the case with the man-made variety. It is this shortening of the corset that can be viewed during the performance of the camel and, indeed, the prime value of the posture at a certain level of competence. With a serious restriction in the range of movement in the diaphragm caused by this shrinkage, the consequences of this are severe but go unnoticed by all physicians of the Western mind-set.

There are many consequences which will be explained. The most profound yet unobservable is the restriction to vena cava articulation. This large blood return pipe passes directly through the diaphragm—it is most interesting to observe that the SUPPLY pipe, the aorta, passes down wards close to the spine and is thus definitely not affected by diaphragm function—and is thus enlarged with each breath. The vena cava has to pass though what is referred to as a hiatus—basically a hole in the diaphragm—but it would have been easy for this pipe to have been placed alongside the supply pipe just as it is in a central heating system. Instead, the vena cava passes though the central part of the diaphragm and it is my contention that the vena cava is heavily influenced by the movement of the diaphragm. With each downward movement of the diaphragm, provided this is accompanied by outwards mobilisation of the ribs, there is inevitably an enlargement of the vena cava, in fact we should call this a distension of the pipe. This action brings with it a reduction in resistance to flow, a reduction in pressure and thus the fluid flow is eased, increasing the volume. This is basic physics, basic fluid behaviour. This must have a direct effect upon the ability of the heart to function as it must upon the general quality of flow throughout the body. If this action so described is working well, then the heart pumps blood around the system and the diaphragm sucks it back—in fact, the diaphragm is acting as a return pump. There is, then, knowledge of what is supposed to happen but this never translates into advice about how one should maintain health. Since this is, in our view, valuable to circulatory health it is a constant source of consternation that amongst "health professionals" generally, there is no talk of proper breathing.

8. Adhesions-external and internal

What is an adhesion? To adhere is to stick to. So adhesions are places where things are sticking together –plainly this occurs where it should not. In fact, what one has to conclude is that every cell, every molecule of the human, indeed of every living thing, is NEVER still. There is always movement—at least that is how it is designed to be. Unfortunately, the human body is hugely tolerant of *immobility*—many of our patients who have presented with moderate pain, have virtually no movement in many spinal joints or the neck or the hips. This is a common experience for fmm practitioners to face in clinic and all those yoga teachers that one speaks to will say a similar thing. But how have so many people got to be like this with so little protest from their bodies?? This is part of our challenge—to understand this phenomenon.

Earlier we referred to the adjoining muscles, the trapezius and rhomboids and erector spinae, each being adjacent to one another. Indeed, they lie in layers and act over the ribs. It is possible for the fmm therapist to actually feel the hardness of adhesion and contracture especially at this place on the body—the whole mass of muscle can be palpated and gradually brought to the point of "normality"—that is soft and pliable. Muscles are supposed to be soft and pliable. They are not efficient if hard and short—hard and short is what if referred to as ***contracture.***

If we continue with this example it is possible to visualise this characteristic and its possible effect. Let us take the erector spinae group of muscles which run from the base of the skull to the sacrum at the bottom of the spine. They are not all in one as it were, but made up of different strands of differing size and girth. But for our purposes it is enough to know that they go north to south. If they contracture, which is the case on at least 70% of the people who come for treatment, the ribs must be affected. It must be that the fascial covering of the ribs known as the periosteum (every bone is covered with periosteum) becomes adherent to the fascial covering of the muscle. The fluid which is suppose to lubricate the surfaces of the fascia—it works well as a lubricant!!—will act as a glue if there is no movement. And how will lack of movement come about??—computer, car, desk-----one of my favourite sayings is that it is not rocket science!! The immobility created by these activities is the usual cause.

 Of course there is usually one bright person who will say that they take plenty of exercise—therefore how could this happen--- indeed many years ago I treated a young woman who had a very severe case of contracture at this part of the body –she was World Windsurfing Champion!!! So –we should be cautious about suggesting that exercise will promote avoidance of contracture since my work with many world class athletes demonstrates that there is as much trouble with them as with couch potatoes!!

The reason it happens is not lack of exercise but lack of contrast in the movement. The erector spinae are designed to move over the ribs when contracting, the rhomboids are designed to move over the erector spinae etc. To become adherent means that this has not happened—there is no other logical conclusion. The same can be palpated at the knee. The iliotibial tract, otherwise known as the tensor fascia lata, runs down the outer part of the thigh and directly influences the function of the knee. If it becomes very tight-that is contractured-it will pull the knee out of running alignment and affect the other muscles of the thigh compounding the problem of incorrect function of the knee. This is a very simple characteristic which can be proven quite simply by stretching the band and then seeing how the gait looks to the eye. In bad cases, especially amongst sportspeople such as hockey players, the band can be felt to be glued to the femur and the head of the fibula. When released the band becomes soft and pliable and the knee runs easily and painlessly. The band can then be felt to be movable on the femur. Of course, this is not something that the average yoga teacher is likely to do although we do in the advanced yoga workshops, promote the checking of this characteristic.

These adhesions appear all over the body, generally where there is very heavy force of muscle contraction. Canoeists are badly affected around the base of the neck. Rowers are badly affected along the thoracic part of the erector spinae. These form what we term severe blockages— blockages to the flow of blood, lymph, energy, as well as to the correct function of the things which they move. The child's shortening hamstrings, visible at the age of 5, are already predisposing it to knee and hip problems in 20 years.

No-one is looking. If pain is reported in teenage—a common scenario— it is usually dismissed as being growing pains. This is incompetence of a high order.

One of the few places where contracture and adhesion has rarely been seen in our clinics is at the bicep and tricep—and this is because this muscle is continually lengthened and tires easily so will complain early. It has been seen on perhaps two canoeists. Otherwise, most parts of the body are affected. From my therapy practice I offer this as the league table of malfunction---in other words the table shows the percentage of people attending my clinic with the stated problem—the problem being my statement of the diagnostic analysis not their symptom statement. It is a crude analysis but serves to indicate the gross.

Most frequent problem---- 90% of people come with C7 and/or L5 seized or almost seized.
Trapezius contracture-----70%
Erector spinae contracture---70%
Thoracic immobility------50%
Hamstring shortening—99%
Hip muscles contractured and joint immobile---25%
Shoulder-bursitis, tendon strain, muscles imbalance 25%
Calf, tibial muscle contracture—20%
If you observe the location of these problems it really means that muscles that are in trouble are anti-gravity muscles—in other words they are posterior and not frontal.
This should not be used as a gospel fact—just a broad indicator

9. Blood Flow Restrictions

In order to understand how blood flows in the human body it is helpful to firstly consider the nature of the flow of fluids. This is a subject usually included in standard school education programmes –certainly at University—for mechanical engineering students.

But if you were studying plumbing this would also be a critical subject for you. Blood is a fluid just as water in your central heating system in your house. There is no fundamental difference in the principles involved in the mechanics of the process of fluid starting at one point and being transported to another via pipework!! See a standard medical chart of the type seen on clinic walls! Consider that there is a readily identifiable network of distribution pipes, starting at the heart and finishing at the return part of the heart. In between there are miles of arteries, arterioles and capillaries for the business of supply of blood and as much to return it to the heart. Just as a pipe system made by man starts off large bore, it ends up small bore, the bore of the pipes being smaller to assist in the maintenance of pressure. If you have to transmit 11 litres of blood per minute from the heart you need a large pipe—this is called the aorta and runs down against the spine until bifurcating in the lower abdomen to serve each leg. The femoral arteries are, thus, smaller since they need to keep up the pressure and of course are only carrying half as much as the main supply pipe. If the pipe size was kept the same then flow would reduce unacceptably in many places because volume was too small.

Central heating systems include a pump---the heart equivalent—but this is where the very simple system in houses loses its comparability. The copper pipes are not elastic—the arteries, arterioles and capillaries are all muscular pipes which act as pumps just like the heart. Similarly, the muscle action of normal everyday activity is the mainstay of this pumping action. So—we have the heart as the primary pumping mechanism, with blood flow being assisted continuously and at every point in the body, by the contraction and relaxation of the vascular pipes and a further action to assist this process of blood distribution being provided by muscle contraction. The pipes are squeezed by the action of muscle thickening and relaxing. We have missed out arguably the most important part of the system—the diaphragm. The role is well documented in nurses anatomy and physiology books but there is no real understanding amongst doctors and specialists—it is ignored in the vascular process despite the role it plays, This is most probably because if the diaphragm fails to work efficiently no one will know. You will not die—so it is dismissed quite easily. Therefore, if you have to undergo heart function assessment via ECG no-one will examine your diaphragm. I call this Internet Knowledge—it is known but not truly ingrained in the consciousness of medics of all persuasions—this includes physiotherapists who one could reasonably say should know. There is no one in the average hospital who truly understands that heart function must be inextricably linked to diaphragm function.

The next bit of understanding required is that each muscular pipe requires—naturally--- a nerve stimulus to enable the contraction and relaxation to occur. Anything which interferes with nerve transmission will have a vascular price tag attached.—there will be some deficiency somewhere. It is, therefore, not enough to look at the pipe work and verify that there are no blockages, a process which vascular surgeons carry out via cameras –the endoscope probe. This will enable the surgeon to observe a real blockage but gives him no understanding as to the quality of flow of blood.

What stimulates the pipe to constrict? This is the sympathetic nervous system—generally the sympathetic system stimulates whilst the parasympathetic relaxes. The nerve stimulus, if the mechanism is functioning correctly, should open the pipes at the appropriate moment and constrict them when needed. We can see in every day function how this works. When you emerge from your centrally heated house into the cold it takes only seconds for your hands to become cold –the sympathetic system has demanded a closure of the capillaries in order to aid in maintaining the core body temperature—we would all consider this to be perfectly normal. But when the spinal nerves are interfered with at any level, this may create either an inappropriate excitation of the sympathetic nerves so that the pipes are closed down when they should be open—or there could be an inhibitory signal which may keep the pipes open when it would be best if they were closed. Much of this incorrect function is the result of inappropriate spinal function—in this section we have dealt with the congestive and inflammatory condition and it is probably these that are responsible for much of what goes wrong in this department. This conclusion is the result of 25 years of treating patients with all manner of mechanical problems of the spine and the major joints rather than purely from the practice of yoga and the observation of the effects of this system.

Now we are able to have a close look at what goes wrong. To do this it is instructive to go back over the fascia and its construction. Let us liken the fascia, especially the superficial fascia, which is the complete wrapping underneath the skin to a complete plastic bag. Now this is highly vascular—there are miles of capillaries embedded along side the nerve endings. The fascia is then a primary defence mechanism. If it becomes contractured, it must affect the vascular workings. A tight muscle must restrict blood flow—blood is the primary carrier for repair materials—the maintenance team depends entirely upon blood flow to enable sufficient nutrient and materials for normal repair to be delivered to all cells. To not provide enough repair materials will create what medics wrongly call "wear and tear". The degraded structures have not worn away—this is especially obvious if one examines the spondylosis in the average middle aged neck which has become immobile for many years and has thus **not** moved so cannot have worn away—they have deteriorated because of lack of nutrient. This is a vastly different notion to that propounded by the average doctor –the average patient aged over 45 complaining of neck stiffness and pain who is otherwise healthy will within minutes of stating the symptoms receive what is laughingly called a diagnosis of------" its probably wear and tear---its your age". The vast majority of patients fitting the description receive just this—with a prescription for anti-inflammatory pills. In itself this is another piece of absurdity-how does anyone know that there is inflammation when the affected structures are at least an inch below the palpating finger. Only inflammation visible and palpable on the surface could accurately be diagnosed. A swollen knee can be seen. Of course, the pill offered as a solution given to get rid of the patient. That is admitted by doctors.

The nature of blood flow restriction is—first and foremost—the presence of immobility. Where ever there is loss of movement there will be reductions in flow. The nature of restriction is loss of mobility –this is the primary—all else stems from this simple fact. That all structures are intended to MOVE –" movement is life, life is movement" This has been stated and restated by many of the most memorable names in physical medicine---Alexander of the Alexander Technique---Moshe Feldendreis, Ida Rolf, Judith Aston.

So neck joints that are not fully mobile will degrade and this degradation is entirely due to shortage of blood flow over years. Naturally, this characteristic is substantially influenced by nutritional quality— degradation is likely to be more significant if one is poorly nourished, which could bring us back to diet!!

 The next important factor is muscle usage and muscle softness. The soft relaxed muscle which has no contracture is best able to permit unimpeded flow of fluids. If contracture occurs then we must consider the effects. Contracture is the progressive shrinkage of the fascia—the fascia adapts its length to the habitual range of movement of muscle. Therefore, unless muscle is regularly stretched there must be contracture. We can look at fascia blood flow, not as we have considered the main arteries and veins as comparable to central heating pipes but as the ditches around the borders of fields all over the countryside. There are million of miles of ditches and these are as important a resource in the management of earth fluid—that is rain!!—as are the rivers. Indeed, the rivers could be seen as the main arteries but the fascia as the less obvious and poor relation of these obvious systems. But they have equal importance—again it is not understood as such by medics. However, farmers DO understand the importance of keeping their ditches clear— they will experience flooding if they are not. Flooding, of course, is the equivalent of congestion—ditches getting over full means congestion is occurring—it is the same principle. Joints of the neck not moving dictates that the arteries and veins serving the ligaments, fascia, joint capsules and little muscles around the joint will be restricted and thus congestion will occur. A further problem will also occur in this situation—the congestion-- which is poor lymph and blood flow through the structures-- will create local nerve irritation. This will, in turn, cause *reflex inhibition* of local muscles. This mean further restrictions in movement. Thus pain creates its own restrictions—nature provides a splint because the local area looks after its own "patch" as it were. The person, therefore, suffers even though she is otherwise healthy, because of this phenomenon of local irritation. For many who fail to resolve this immobility—there will simply be a further reduction in spinal mobility and eventually they will truly manifest what was said at the initial consultation-"its your age". This statement condemns many to early immobility.

If you were to examine the arterial and venous pathways around the human neck, you would see a hugely complex network of pipes, most having a tortuous route around the vertebrae. If the neck is not extended and flexed and rotated, the pipes will not be required to move. Many of these pipes have many bends –indeed, the pipe routes are rather like the map of the Swiss Alps—hair pin bends everywhere. The potential for congestion is massive. It is almost as though the neck especially cries out for mobilisation—and we present this as the evidence of such a demand!

Let us now take a further serious restriction—compression from various causes. We should take as our first port of call—sitting! The hamstrings are –in modern times—under constant compression from sitting—there is a vascular effect. Currently there is much talk of deep vein thrombosis—airlines are especially targeted. This is another medical absurdity—as though sitting for a few hours is the cause of this problem. It is not-but it is a long period of sitting that will bring it out-but it would happen anyway but perhaps in a different way. Let us look at what is happening. Take a cross section—cut through—the thigh. Imagine looking down on this section having cut it right through—you will see that the arteries and veins run between the fascial clefts. These are the separate wrappings around each of the muscle bellies in the thigh. If the thigh fascia is contractured then there will be a thickening of the muscle belly and a shortening of the muscle overall. This means that the pipes running through the muscles are subjected to more compression than would be the case if there were normal length of muscle. Add to this the effect of sitting—for the average person that will mean about 7 stone resting on just the hamstrings and gluteals—and it is obvious that further compression must take place. This can be felt by the sensitive yoga practitioner to be the case—leg blood flow restriction can actually be felt. We now have, thus, fascial shrinkage pressing on the pipes throughout their entire length as well as gravitional effects—direct force of compression. This is, in our view, the primary reason why hamstrings are universally short, from the age of about 5—whereas the quadriceps which are on top of the thigh are never shortened. It should now be possible to see that exercise does not solve these problems. Yoga does but exercise does not—indeed, only those activities that actively stretch tissue and plastically deform it will be able to solve the problems caused by fascial shrinkage. And the vast majority of yoga participants when first appearing in a yoga class are in this category. I have in 20 years of teaching taught several thousand people and have only a couple of times seen someone who was flexible and thus had no substantial fascial shrinkage. 99% of people that I see in classes—and this goes for all those people that I have taught yoga who have become teachers themselves—are fascially contractured, usually badly. The ignorance of this simple fact is universal—doctors, nurses, midwives, health visitors, surgeons, consultant orthopaedic specialists, as well as osteopaths and chiropractors—they are all ignorant of this and it is probably the root of all the really poor diagnosis I have seen in over 20 years of treating patients. So many of these patients have been the rounds looking for a cure.

Now we have a complete list –in summary-of all those elements that contribute to restrictions in blood flow. When blood flow is mentioned we should also include lymph since the rules are similar although the pipework is much less obvious. Not all lymph is transported by pipe. There is primarily fascial shrinkage. There is then joint immobility. This affects the quality and quantity of joint lubricant—synovial fluid. Congestion leads to nerve irritation and this causes further restrictions in movement. We have direct compression and lack of stretching of structures which would cause easing of flow if it were performed. There is then neurological interference which prevents proper signals from being sent to arteries and veins and spurious signals will either inhibit the opening of an artery to stimulate more flow or it could restrict it just by over stimulation. This over- stimulation could be the result of nerve irritation caused by congestion or immobility or trauma or direct compression.

There is thus a continuous maintaining cycle from which there is no escape except by stretching. This is the knowledge gained by the yogis thousands of years ago. Despite such amazing systemic knowledge there remains massive ignorance. I hope this book may help to lift the cloak preventing proper understanding.

At this point it could be helpful to you to reproduce a few sentences from a very old booklet produced for a gathering of French osteopaths many years ago. The booklet was written by John Wernham who was taught osteopathy by Littlejohn who was one of Andrew Taylor Still's students over a hundred years ago and is widely regarded as the father of osteopathy.

"Therefore the osteopathic idea is not that of a bone lesion but the change in biological characteristics which must be discussed, diagnosed and treated from the standpoint of mobility. In line with this the foundation on which all the vitality of the body is built is stimulation so that stimulation and inhibition osteopathy are the ways and means of dealing with the body from the biological standpoint because in the cyclical movements of the body theses are the two aspects of the vital activity of the organs and tissues. Disease is either the result of too much or too little stimulation.

All this is based upon the four cardinals—flexion, extension side bending and rotation. Any form of corrective technique that ignores thee fundamentals will gain results in more by luck than judgement and desirable and complete physiological changes will not be made adequately."

I realise that here we are discussing yoga and not osteopathy but it is clear from much of his writing that he did not accept the yank and wrench mechanism which he states are "slick Americanism" but believed in the gradual improvement of the whole organism. He could have been describing yoga!

10 Muscle Strength

Muscle strength is a function of many factors. We are concerned here with what goes wrong with the average human frame. In this regard, muscle strength is affected mostly by poor neurological transmission—in other words nerves are usually compressed or poorly served nutritionally and thus do not send their signals as well as they would if there were no interference. This interference is due usually to the processes described so far-we can sum up this by using the term fascial contracture. But there is another very poorly understood characteristic—that the short muscle does not permit firing of all nerve stimuli; this means that the shorter the muscle the smaller the number of muscle fibres that will be made available to contract and thus do the work requested. Now the body is very clever so it does not let the owner know such a thing—only perhaps by tiring the muscle quicker than might be the case. The power of the muscle is not, therefore, entirely dependent upon the size of the muscle. It is as much dependent upon the quality of nerve stimulus which in turn is a function of how soft, long and relaxed is the muscle. The long relaxed muscle permits 100% of the fibres to function so that each fibre does not become overloaded. The short muscle has less than the full compliment working and thus will have less strength as well as less work capacity. This will also dictate that each fibre has more work to do.

The usual way that muscle fibres rest is that blocks of fibres do some work and then rest while another set of blocks of fibres takes over. If the muscle receives a demand for 100% strength then all the fibres will do the job and thus the muscle will tire very quickly. If many fibres are not functioning properly then it is not difficult to see that efficiency is what suffers. If this is, say, at the gastrocnemius—the calf—then snapping of the tendon may result. This is fairly common today.

All those attending yoga classes and demonstrating fascial shortening—the vast majority—are thus not getting their potential strength out of muscle. The tight muscle also consumes more energy than the soft relaxed muscle-so the process of stretching should reduce inefficiency. Blood flow must also affect the strength of muscle since a great deal of blood has to be pumped to muscle in order to make it function.

11. Mechanical Dysfunction

We are here considering what are the human problems and how they occur. Mechanical dysfunction is probably the most frequent imposition on the human being, especially in Western culture. Let us take a common condition and examine this. You are a teenager. You are riding a horse and you incur a fall off the horse. After a couple of days you have recovered from the effects—bruising has declined, pain has reduced— this is the aftermath of a fall when there is bound to be bruising and perhaps some tearing of tissue. During a fall, I believe that the body's primal instinct is to tighten up all muscle around the spinal column in order to preserve the spinal nerves. This is the worst case scenario for any human body—spinal cord injury—so the body has its own inbuilt mechanism to avoid this. The whiplash effect of a car accident is a typical example of when the primal instinct for preserving the spinal cord shows itself most frequently. When treating patients who have had whiplash, always there is massive muscle spasm in evidence. Joints of the spine are always thus badly seized up whilst accidents never affect shoulder joints even though these may have been the primary site of injury. Hence the theory put forward—we do not however have any irrefutable proof!

You are now operating again (back to our 11 year old) without pain but unknown to you two joints of the upper thorax are not moving properly. You are not able to turn your body fully –but this is not detected because it is seldom that this characteristic will be challenged in normal life. If you are competing in a demanding sport it is likely that you will eventually experience pain—if you were to visit an fmm practitioner then mechanical dysfunction would be palpated. We, therefore, define mechanical dysfunction as those set of circumstances in the human frame that impose a limit upon normal function. An inability to turn the neck fully may be detected by a driver used to reversing with the whole body turned in the car seat. This is a common example of how older people detect the presence of substantial neck rotation restriction—they come to a junction whilst driving and find that the neck limitation of range will not permit them to see round a difficult bend—so they twist the thorax as well. This is the most common example of mechanical dysfunction. Less common would be the hip joint that has been x-rayed and no degradation detected that starts to cause its owner to limp and to stop walking after short distances. Here mechanical dysfunction has created pain which is the natural way of the body saying that it does not wish for the owner to use the hip for walking in case the deterioration (which has not been detected on an x-ray because this method only picks up GROSS pathology) leads to more degradation. This is another example of just how poor the average GP is at diagnosis since many of our patients have pain and come with their x-ray results which show clearly that there is "nothing wrong with the hip joint". These immortal words! The examination is almost never backed up by any physical examination which would easily and quickly show loss of joint range. It is a simple test that takes about 5 seconds to perform—it is not done. The patient is dismissed with the words " there is nothing wrong" ringing loudly in his ears—of course there is little point in his saying that how can the pain be explained because he will just be offered pain killers. Most thinking people are very unhappy with this notion.

We can say with reasonable conviction that there are two routes to mechanical dysfunction—the first is long term decline of mobility and the second is trauma. Of course we have to be willing to consider that diseases like TB or rheumatoid arthritis will also create mechanical dysfunction by restricting joint range. But we will adhere to that aspect of human life that we very well understand—the former two sources - since we see these in droves!!

So now let us consider another mechanism—the skier who has a fully functioning knee that has no problem. Descending a steep piste, she gets one ski caught and one knee is badly strained. This is a genuine strain— the circumstance in which a joint is suddenly and forcibly placed outside its design range of movement. The internal ligaments are overstretched- genuinely strained-and the woman is plastered in a hospital or at least has a mechanical clamp applied to her knee to prevent movement whilst healing takes place. This of course can be considered a genuine injury— pain does not dictate an injury since neck joints becoming tight and creating pain is not a strain and the meaning of the pain is very different from the strained knee joint. The strained knee joint demands to be **immobilised**—the pain has to be interpreted in this way. But the seized joint of the neck which also creates pain, demands to be **mobilised**. This difference creates many diagnostic problems for therapists especially for physiotherapists whose general inclination has always been to suggest rest. Indeed, many of the World Class athletes that I have treated over the past 20 years have come for treatment following weeks of enforced rest— the rest has not produced any improvement in the condition, a predictable outcome for the vast majority. There is thus a simple rule which we could invent—the chronic problem demands mobilisation regardless. The recent injury to tissue demands a short period of restricted use just to allow repair to take place. Mobilisation should begin after no more than a few weeks. For most injuries this should be a few

DAYS not weeks!! If there is no fracture detected on an x-ray then I will almost always begin by massaging the area to get energy and blood flow stimulated and usually three sessions is sufficient to get even the bad case back to normal when most would have propose rest taking months rather than days to recover. Nature needs help!!

The skier has injured the knee –it is strapped up and now the strapping has been removed the person will begin to use it. For most fit healthy people there will be a complete recovery from the "injury" part of the problem. What we discover in clinic is that, in the case of the knee injury, there is tensor fascia lata adherence, calf muscle contracture, hamstring adherence to the femur, knee cap malfunction due to misalignment and sometimes the quadriceps have contracture. This latter is very rare but these are the circumstances in which it is most likely to have been created. The patient or yoga student coming years after the ski-ing accident, reports knee pain that has no specific origin and often the person has forgotten what has originally created the problem—they don't link the history since they follow what the medic says which is that after one year or more there should be no more pain because the injury will have cleared up. Another example of poor understanding of the nature of injury. Of course the injured tissue will have repaired—but the legacy is malfunction. Malfunction is not injury and thus there is nothing to "heal". The knee will be malfunctioning as a result of the distortions in the fascia, which in turn are making the knee rolling surfaces malalign during use. This is hard to see or to detect in any other way—it is possible to see patterns during yoga postures but it is very unlikely that even a good podiatrist would pick this up.

The frozen shoulder is further evidence of mechanical dysfunction although it may have traumatic origins just like the knee in our previous example.

The spinal vertebral immobility probably causes most of the dysfunctions in the human body—if there are, for example, two upper thoracic vertebrae which are not moving they are capable of creating inhibition to scapula movement as well as pain on moving. But the yoga teacher in a class of stiff people gets the best lesson in mechanical dysfunction with each class. What the participants are being asked to perform is a series of postures which all children can perform with ease. In other words yoga postures are the most effective way for the human being to bring herself back to full mechanical function—thus removing dysfunctional elements. Largely yoga can do this but sometimes it is necessary for the person to have physical therapy just to "blast out "the worst of the problems.

It should be plain what we mean by mechanical dysfunction, from the preceding descriptions. Unfortunately we live in times when medics strive to label groups of symptoms and it would seem that this is considered adequate, obviating the need for any physical examination. Here is a very recent case. An 11 year old boy is labelled as dyspraxic and dyslexic. He is presented as a patient and complains that his feet hurt. He has been given another label by a GP —Severs disease. This is reputedly similar to the label Osgood –Schlatter—the bony growth plates in the growing body are somehow not working properly. Medics have been happy with this label for many years despite the ease with which the experienced practitioner can treat the cause—invariably short hamstrings and contractured quadriceps. The boy in question can locate the moment foot pain occurred—he ran along a ploughed field. On examination he could be seen –it is very obvious-that he has fallen arches in both feet. The feet are not quite flat but this is not far away. He has been using orthotics for years to help prevent malfunction of knees and hips. No-one had bothered to consider the reason he put forward, no-one had examined his hamstrings which were so short that he could not touch his knees. His calves were heavily contractured—the combination of these two factors is more than enough to justify stretching both. Now in this case, no amount of understanding of yoga could make his feet "normal", any more than a woman with a foot bunion could be made to have feet that looked pretty. The bunnionated foot will always malfunction, permitting the big toe to roll inwards towards the other toes, eventually squeezing the space for the other toes. One could assist by recommending sandals or square ended shoes that do not squeeze the toes but this does not change the fact that the feet will always work according to this restriction. In the same way the boy with fallen arches will always walk in a manner that creates a compensatory device. We would still refer to this phenomenon as mechanical dysfunction but we could easily split into two sections those dysfunctions that can be restored and those that cannot. Thus, it is preferable to see our 11 year old as having two mechanical dysfunctions—the first is contractured muscle which can easily be solved, spinal joints which do not move well—this can also easily be solved—and then flattening arches which cannot be solved, but can be assisted. The latter can be assisted by orthotics and treatment but not obviously and directly by yoga.

We leave this section, reiterating the concept that mechanical dysfunction in the majority that enter yoga is created by contracture of myofascial structures—short muscles—and stiff spinal joints. The *primary* problem is muscle shortening and eventual contracture. And the reason for contracture is the *lack of understanding of the need to prevent it.*

In this regard it has similarities with dental decay—of course, nowadays the great majority understand what needs to be done with this—but the level of ignorance of the origin of stiffness is universal. In 25 years of professional therapy practice I have come across only a handful of folk who analysed their problems as having the origin in loss of muscle range. Statistically that amounts to around 0.1%.

12. Disease and Pathology

What problems occur within the human species could be separated into sections. There are those viral and bacterial in origin and plainly our concern when discussing yoga is not with these although all those practising yoga would contend that their overall health has improved since beginning yoga.

We could then move to the opposite end of the spectrum of causes and specify the diseases of consumption—these are readily identifiable as not being things "you just catch". Obesity, cardiovascular pathology—heart disease especially, atherosclerosis (hardening of the arteries), arthritis and arthrosis, rheumatoid arthritis, diabetes —of course the list is much more extensive than just these few. We illustrate these because it is the diseases of consumption, as they are referred to in the holistic health world, which are those things which come as a result of conspicuous lifestyle choices. The causes generally considered to be the most common are, lack of dietetic nutrient, excessive sedentary work, low level of exercise, too much stress, lack of exercise and carrying too much weight. Holistic therapists would also include the high level of chemicals polluting the food, "electro-smog" as excessive radio waves is known, density of vehicle traffic, supermarket shopping and a few less obvious.

Within the list of diseases of consumption also come the cancers which many believe are the result of the same factors. It is harder to trace the origin since many of the affected people are what would have been classified as fit and healthy—not overweight and well –off financially, so not having to work too hard,--and eating well. This is very difficult for some to consider that what they have classified as a good diet—generous portions of green veg and fruit—had not been adequate to protect them from cancer. So it has been dismissed by many cancer sufferers as irrelevant—they have failed to thoroughly examine the origin of their food and seen that much of it probably originated in the fields of Lincolnshire which have been discovered to be virtually devoid of nutrient. The American nutritionist Dr John Wallack who dissected more humans after death than any other living person, and who dissected more dead animals than anyone else simply states that the state of diseased tissue for all diseased people and animals can be seen to be the result of lack of nutrient. He has adequate nutritional research as well as having the evidence of pathological examination to back up his findings---he has needless to say, been dismissed by the food lobby as a crank. Inconvenient truths are regularly dismissed by the "authorities" who have public access to media coverage as well as a fervent belief in themselves.

When we use the word pathology we use it in the sense of their being something wrong with a person—we use it as a short hand statement for the words" the existence of pathological change in the body". By this we mean to transmit that the person can be found to have some identifiable problem which doctors could find on the many tests which are carried out in the average hospital. What we mean by mechanical malfunction has been explained but reiteration here would be useful for comparison—and for this we can return to our man with hip pains who had x-rays which clearly show no bony deterioration in his hip joints and no loss of space between the ball and the socket—thus by implication the cartilage would be in good order. His GP declared that he had nothing wrong with his hip joints—but what was found in our clinic was massive shortening of all the soft tissues around the joint, creating an inability to flex and internally rotate the joints. So **pathologically** he was well but **functionally** he was in a poor state. The poor functional state would eventually lead to loss of cartilage which would then create deterioration of bony quality at the ball and socket because this is the mechanism that usually dictates pathological change—first appears the loss of mobility and functional quality because there is shortening of soft tissue structures and the consequent reduction in fluid transmission. Then comes the "wear and tear" –again we state that this is the wrong wording. The wear as it is called is not wear at all –it is degeneration caused by lack of proper movement.

 Interestingly this man has been attending yoga classes for several weeks after coming to see me for treatment and already the pains he was experiencing have reduced dramatically. Pain emanating from worn joints would not go away so readily—but if it did decrease it would, from experience, take many years of patient and dedicated self-help.

At this point I propose to include the writings of several therapists who have detailed the pathological changes that have been seen to have taken place when dissecting dead bodies. Symptom description allied to post mortem findings has, as a mechanism, enabled the medical investigator to see what he considers the reason for symptoms.

Here, then, is a series of statements from various published sources which I include as though they all appeared together. These are rather abrupt and terse not because this is how they appear in the publications but because I have simply extracted the "meaty" substance and left all the peripheral explanation. I am sure that in so doing I have not in any way distorted the message that the writer had given since I have read the whole publication before making such extraction.

Ashmore, E. *Osteopathic Mechanics*
Tamor Pierston Publishers, London, 1981.

"Injuries to ligaments either precede or accompany injuries to the discs. Hyperflexion strains in the lumbar spine have been shown to damage the supraspinous and interspinous ligaments first, then the capsular ligaments and then the disc. The supraspinous and interspinous ligaments are invariably ruptured or slack in patients with a disc prolapse."

"The circumferential tears are commonly thought to be caused by repetitive rotation strains. Because of the orientation of the annular fibres, during axial rotation only half of them are able to resist the movement, the outer fibres being stretched more then the inner ones."

"A disc prolapse involves the displacement of nuclear material. It is most common between the age of 30 and 50, after which the nuclei have become more fibrotic and less likely to overload. There is less likelihood for the nuclear material to be expressed as a semifluid substance since there is drying out taking place with age.

A prolapse can either be

1. An annular protrusion –when displaced nuclear material stretches the outer annulus, causing it to bulge outwards—in this case the annulus is not completely ruptured.

2. A nuclear extrusion when pulp escapes from the disc through a ruptured annulus.

"Gradual prolapse is the most common of the failings. The annular lamellae probably start out as distorted forming radial fissures. Nuclear pulp then breaks through the distorted lamellae causing the outermost lamellae and the adhering posterior longitudinal ligament to protrude. Because of the insidious nature of events leading up to the prolapse, the "final straw" which gives rise to the patients signs and symptoms may be caused by a trivial event like bending to pick up a piece of paper. Activities in life which could lead to the gradual disc prolapse are those involving repetitive bending and lifting, not necessarily in the flexed position. This type of prolapse is often preceded by bouts of lumbar pain which the patient passes off as "muscular". It is possible that one of the causes of this symptomology is distortion of the outer fibres which are innervated.

"In order for healing to occur following trauma or degeneration of an intervertebral disc, a good blood supply is necessary. The very outermost layers of a normal disc are penetrated by blood vessels and so, theoretically, circumferential tears could have a chance to heal. Following trauma or as a natural process of ageing, blood vessels penetrating the end plates and the annulus, and fresh granulation tissue invading the nucleus, have been seen at surgery and they provide evidence of a healing process. Initial healing by scar formation may have sufficiently different characteristics to produce a change in the mechanical behaviour of the annulus. Insufficient evidence exists of the rate of turnover of collagen in human beings—experiments suggest it is likely to be extremely slow."

"The nerve roots can be compressed along their course through the spinal canal, radicular canals or in the intervertebral foramina. The most common cause of nerve root compression in the lumbarspine is the disc, either from bulging or from an extrusion of nuclear material. However, it is by no means the only cause—osteophyte formation, spondylolithesis, hypertrophied lagamentum spinal stenosis or other pathological lesions are possible causes."

"Where the spinal canal is large, the likelihood of cord compression is very much reduced. In the cervical region, the average diameter of the spinal canal is 17mm with 10 mm the average cord diameter. Therefore gross changes in the canal dimensions need to be present before cord compression could reasonably be seen to be possible. However, in persons with spondylosis it seems to be more common that the spinal canal suffers stenosis or narrowing to the point where the average measurement was seen to be 14mm making cord compression more likely"

"Once a mass of nuclear material has been extruded from the disc, it becomes possible for detachment of movement along the nerve root migrating some distance from the disc."

"The decisive factor in the production of symptoms and signs is the available space. The cauda equina and its blood vessels are often compromised to a greater extent than individual spinal nerves."

"Incidence of arthrosis---with repetitive stresses over years a chronic synovial reaction becomes established and a synovial fold projects into the joint space between articular surfaces. Fragments of cartilage may break of forming loose bodies which can lie freely in the joint or become attached to the synovial membrane. Simultaneously, changes to the capsule can occur, creating a dense mat further restricting movement.

Oliver, J and Middleditch, A. 1991 *Functional Anatomy of the Spine.* Butterworth and Heinemann, Oxford.

Here is an extract from the world famous Dr James Cyriax, spine surgeon.

"All joints that contain intra-articular cartilage are apt to suffer from internal derangement. Small pieces of cartilage become detached and then displaced. This is a very common event at any spinal joint." Now contrast this with another very logical step which this man takes –and this is on the subject of stretching the capsule of a joint

"When the thick strong capsule of a joint needs to be stretched out, the quick movement that serves to break adhesions is inappropriate for it merely hurts the patient and leads to further muscle resistance. To stretch out a tough structure—i.e. the capsule of a hip joint or a shoulder joint, requires the long steady push maintained for as long as the patient can stand it—say a minute."

J .Cyriax. Bailliere Tindall
Textbook Of Orthopaedic Medicine
1983. London

This is most interesting because it is the closest that any surgeon I have heard of has got to yoga. Is this not precisely what we are about in our yoga? Of course, those fmm practitioners will also recognise that this is what I have taught them—that slow stretching of structures is superior to high velocity thrusts so beloved of those with whom my early experiences were acquired—the osteopaths. It also helps the fmm practitioner to understand why their many patients, who have complained about ineffective osteopathy and chiropractic, have not improved with manipulation but have recovered rapidly with fmm which has included slow stretching and is thus strongly aligned with yoga.

It is also of interest to me because over the past 5 years of physical therapy practice I have sent hundreds of patients for MRI scans for suspected disc herniations and have not yet come across one of the reports which states that there is a piece of disc broken off and is pressing against the nerve root. All those positive tests—and this is all but about three—indicated disc prolapse in all the possible stages of degeneration from the mildest bulge to the complete extrusion—but never a loose body so beloved of Dr Cyriax. I have no idea why this is so since I have immense respect for the work of this one man and who has operated on thousands of people so should know just how many of the symptoms are due to nerve root compression caused by piece of disc. It, of course, could be that the piece of disc is so small that it does not show up well on the MRI –but having studied many MRI's this seems unlikely. I must add that the MRI scans I receive have all been studied by Consultant Radiologists, several of them, so missing something like this is unlikely. But I have no explanation for this.

What is interesting about all the one-liners above is that the human disc and its associated structures must be seen as a potential mine-field for trouble!

What is most interesting about the research work for all researchers is that focuses exclusively on the local condition and does not offer any discussion on the subject of INITIAL CAUSE. If for no other reason, this book is important since I feel that we as yoga and fmm practitioners can find acceptable answers for our students and patients because we fundamentally believe that for the majority of healthy people the cause is loss of mobility. Thus restoration of mobility with yoga inevitably produces an overall increase in health which has to have its by-product in the spinal pathology. The regular allusion to the healing process also encourages one to persuade more people to take up yoga despite all that may have been said to them by others----namely that their spinal condition is incurable. I have no personal knowledge of blood vessels serving ligaments close to spinal discs but all the research work I have read states there is no healing mechanism in the disc itself—confirmed by Adams and co.—but that the presence of extensive vascularity around the annular/ligamentous junction implies that disc healing will take place. I do not know if this is credible but it is when you understand the nature of the disc and its replenishment mechanism that you can accept that, as a unit designed for horizontal function, lack of adequate blood supply to the disc itself is not so much a human failing as inappropriate adaptation to the upright position. Indeed, this notion is central to my view that we are poorly adapted to two legs and that this is entirely why yoga was invented. In the horizontal position the spinal vertebrae are subjected to negligible stress and loading is identical at all points.

Returning to the theme earlier, surely it must be obvious that yoga postures daily stretch the joints and their capsules and thus prevent loss of motion which in turn, prevents degeneration???? The movement of all spinal vertebrae daily will guarantee that degeneration of a local nature will not occur—of course it is still possible to encounter global degeneration in the case of disease and poor diet which are unlikely to be seriously influenced –at least so obviously –by the practices of yoga although in my experience the whole health of the individual improves with yoga.

The point I wish to make after including all this research data provided by physios, is that it is another example of how local thinking is the dominant mechanism—it at no time stimulates the researcher or indeed the physio, to consider what might be the STARTING POINT FOR DISORDER. It seems not to create in the individual the urge to find out—students of yoga generally find themselves burning with this urge to know how and why—but it is plain that this characteristic is very rare.

I propose to round off this section by quoting from Robin McKenzie's The Lumbar Spine, another book I bought decades ago. Equally I never read the introduction which is now, once again, most revealing about the mind –set of the physiotherapist.

"Low back pain is not necessarily a consequence of degenerative processes for many patients with recurring low back pain have no evidence of degenerative changes and patients with clear evidence of pathological change do not have back pain. (I would add here that this was written before MRI scans were available so what does not show on an x-ray could easily be visible on the former.) The incidence of occupational back pain is the same for manual workers as for sedentary workers the difference being that the former cannot work with the pain and take time off. (Again this may not be so simple as stated since manual labourers may not feel the same sense of oppression by employer nor perhaps the same sense of dedication that is often associated with middle-class well motivated well-paid white collar workers. I stress this is not my language!!"

 He goes on." If the problems surrounding low back pain were as simple as that there would be little need for clinicians and therapists to devote so much time to its treatment. However, the difficulties do not lie in treating a particular episode of low back pain but more in the prevention of future episodes. From my own figures it appears that about 62% of patients attending for treatment have had episodic pain on at least three occasions in the past 5 years. Although self-limiting, low back pain will often recur and the recurrences tend to become progressively more severe with each successive attack. If we are to succeed in reducing the incidence of low back pain we must aim our treatments at patient education and teaching of preventive methods. Therefore treatment must be implemented during an attack of pain. A patient who has no pain cannot be taught effectively to stop the pain." This is the most extraordinary assertion!!

He goes on to make many logical points.

"Posture greatly affects back pain. Sitting slumped will produce ligament pain which will be difficult to disguise when rising. Studies in 1972 and 1979 found that 75 and 87% of people reporting back pain had a loss of lumbar extension (back bending) and in affluent societies man gradually loses the ability to perform certain movements. From my own observations it seems that those reaching age 30 have already lost a good deal of lumbar extension. As this loss increases the patient will be forced to walk slightly more stooped. The third predisposing factor is lumbar flexion—the average sedentary worker does not perform a lumbar extension after childhood, spending all working and relaxing times bent forward."

McKenzie writes his whole book around the notion that the disc bulges or herniates and this state is only aided by the process of forced extension. In other regards his influences by Dr Cyriax are obvious and accurate and in line with principles of engineering. Then he also comes tantalisingly close to seeing what has happened from childhood. It is perhaps their misfortune that they have seemingly spent no time in the presence of little children because if they had it would be plain that full movement is lost by the age of 15 and it is a long and gradual loss from then on till the stoop of old age so beloved of all writers on the subject.

It may already be apparent that just within the small number of books that I posses, there are numerous mentions which lead the thinker into the realm now approaching. But there is one other influence worth including—this is a selection of snippets from a book on pathology written by a professor of Histopathology in a London hospital. He launches straight in with his introductory sentence that when a person becomes ill, the symptoms are due to a disturbance of the normal functions of some of the cells of the body and he goes on to say that it is the business of pathology to study these disturbed functions and structural changes, to learn how they arise, how they progress and how they affect other cell system. He says   it also takes account of factors which restore the changes to normal. The work of the Italian dissectors of the 16th Century showed that clinical signs and symptoms could be related to underlying lesions found at post mortem. The subsequent use of the microscope clarified the nature of many of these lesions and led to the development of the concepts of organ and cell pathology. Fortunately he goes on to say that virtually every disease has a multifactorial origin, genetic endowment and environmental influences playing their part. Factors such as poverty, poor food, overcrowding, malnutrition, polluted water, all play their part.

At this point he goes off into the details of pathology and the whole book leaves behind that still small voice---"It is the business of pathology to study these disturbed functions and structural changes, to learn how they arise"---------------. I am still trying to find some explanation—how do they arise? What is explained is the WHAT but never the HOW, except that HOW is interpreted as the progression of local cell degeneration, and not my meaning which would simply be ORIGIN----- what started it all going down hill??? No answers are provided—and other authors follow suit in their explanations.

13. The Laws Governing Function

There is one simple "law" which I termed many years ago which I feel still holds true for the vast majority of circumstances.—
--every joint should be capable of moving through its full range of movement at will. If it is not then symptoms may ensue

This should not truly require any further explanation if you have read this far. But just in case let us spell it out as plainly as we know how. If you watch a 5 year old lying face down and then ask her to bend backwards you will see that there is a 180degree movement of the spine. This is normal-this is the design range!! Take a 30 year old and ask that the same movement be performed and you will see that there is less than half this range, often it will be a 70% loss. The person has, thus, functional loss of a very high order and some pathological result is inevitable—it is usually back trouble!!

There is one obstacle to the logic of this first law and it is this; muscles move joints. Therefore, to be utterly logical it is essential to consider that if a joint is not moving through its full range this must be the consequence of either the person simply not taking the joint through this range OR the full range is not available—this dictates that the muscles are not able to move the joint through its full range or that the person is not able to move joints through their full range because of the constraining restrictions of muscle length—this is referred to as myofascial contracture. Hence our corollary to the first law—or it could be the 2nd Law of Function

All muscles should be capable of being lengthened to their full design length—if any muscle is not so capable then it will produce some effect. The effect most commonly will be loss of range of a joint or pain resulting from contracture.

Our contention is that all minor pathology of the spine, such as spondylosis, results from this loss of movement.

The first Law of Function then should really be that which we have here called the 2nd Law—and the second should really be the first. We have left it as we have stated because the realisation of the truth of the two laws did not fully dawn until after what we have called the first was fully explained—so we have chosen to leave it as it is because this is how it is explained in so much of our existing literature. In any event it is sufficient to state that all joints and muscles should be capable of being moved through their full range if symptoms are to be avoided-this adequately covers all possibilities.

Here, then, we have our first major law of function. Osteopaths have their law as Structure Governs Function and Function Governs Structure and this will now be explained because it also has much to offer anyone wishing to understand why things go wrong.

The simplest example can be seen in the upright 5 year old child. If you took an x-ray of the spine it would be revealed that the shape is the classical double S shape. If the person grows up retaining this same upright posture then the vertebrae in the rib cage will each have parallel top and bottom. If as a teenager the young person starts to stoop and retains the neck inclination that results, into the twenties when bony development and growth finish, the vertebrae will adapt to the forces imposed and become wedge –shaped, with the front being narrower than the rear. Now if the person tries to become fully upright as they were at age 5, it will be found to be impossible because the shape of the bones is dictating the postural inclination. Thus, at first the way the spine works dictates what shape it will be—function governs structure------- but when the vertebrae are wedge shaped the structure will be seen to be governing the method of working for the whole spine-structure governs function.

These are the very obvious elements of functional law. Now let us take a common scenario, a problem regularly presenting in our clinics. The 55 year old woman arrives with a very painful neck which she cannot move in any direction. Up until last week she was pain free and the neck was normal—that is her statement. It transpires that the results of an MRI scan two years ago showed spondylotic change in the neck vertebrae. Now there is the possibility that the minor degeneration will create minor irritation if the neck is challenged. Her report is she has done nothing unusual but has had several long aircraft flights during which she fell asleep in awkward positions. Neck range restriction has not been created by fascial shrinkage but by painful inhibition—the natural response to pain is for the area to become splinted—the natural response has been for the minor irritation to cause a splint to occur and it is this which has created loss of range of movement. It is not fascial shrinkage, nor is it just loss of range of movement of the neck vertebrae because in our example the woman had got full range of movement before she left the country.

There is a common further law. A 45 year old man has run a lot for pleasure. He now limps badly –he has had x-rays and there is no break, no bony abnormality. The joints of the foot are normal in range but the tibial compartment muscles are very hard. Working these muscles removes the pain and the person can now walk normally and run again. This is a functional abnormality of the muscles of the lower leg which has created inhibition causing the man to limp. This has no pathological content and would not appear on any test known to medicine-it can only be discovered by feel.

There appeared earlier in Part One an analysis of fascial contracture. The fundamental law governing the behaviour of this ubiquitous material can be simply stated—unless you lengthen it, it will adapt in length to the range of movement habitually used by the muscle. We can say that this is the foundation of all malfunctions in the human frame and that this is the origin of the yoga system of postures –each posture will stretch the fascia until the range is regained.

In fact it would be wise to give the above another title—Law No 3

Fascia is relatively inelastic so that it will adapt to the habitual range of use engaged in each muscle. Eventually if the pattern of muscle use is maintained then contracture occurs which effectively dictates a limitation of movement in the part in question. This is a simple law and its implication is that unless you stretch each muscle then the fascia will adapt itself to the habitual range of use.

14. Neurological Implications

The nervous system is divided, roughly speaking, into sensory and motor components. The sensory are those which carry impulses to the brain and the motor nerves carry impulses from the brain back to the muscles and various organs. The sensory system is served by two types of receptors, the exteroceptive and the interoceptive The former, as implied by the name, receive stimuli from the world around us and are present in the eyes, ears, nose, mouth, skin and mucous membranes. With their help we recognise touch, temperature, taste, smell and pain and we are able to see and to hear.

The interoceptors are situated in the deeper strata—such as muscles, tendons, joints, organs, blood vessels, the internal ear and so on. They are constantly supplying the lower brain centres with information on the positions of various parts of the body relative to each other, and on the state of tension of various muscles and tendons.

The neuromuscular or motor system has a dual nature—phasic and tonic. Of these two the phasic component is more obvious and more easily observable. The movements of the eyeballs, the swinging of the arms or the movement of the legs when walking are all phasic movements. But it is the tonic reaction which not only forms the background for phasic reaction but also sustains or inhibits it. The interoceptive-tonic mechanism does not impinge on the conscious. In general, the exteroceptive impulses excite the phasic reactions (which are passing) while the interoceptive impulses regulate the tonic reactions. It is important to remember that while the phasic movement is momentary, involving a group of muscles, the interoceptive –tonic mechanism is continuous and diffuse and provides at all times the means by which phasic movements are possible.

The muscle tone is only part of the much larger whole. The integrated phenomenon in modern physiological psychological terminology is known as "postural substrate". The word postural is not the rather narrow definition of how erect you are but the whole package of how you behave and move --and just BE. In the normal organism the postural substrate has to be in continuously dynamic and fluid state, constantly varying as the body demands. Yoga teaches that by attacking the abnormal postural substrate and reconditioning it to its previous adaptable and dynamic state, modification of the emotional state can be achieved providing mental tranquillity.

The neuromuscular system is so composed that for every group of muscles that go into contraction, another group undergoes relaxation. In states of mental tension, this reciprocal innervation becomes defective. The reflex inhibition normally permitting relaxation to occur is interfered with to the extent that movement is inhibited. This is what eventually creates the state of muscle contracture—the permanent state of hardness in muscle. Asanas, by their very nature, create a mechanism to remove this contracture and thus eventually the naturally occurring mechanism of reciprocal inhibition is restored.

What are the major difficulties thrown up by the normal problems facing humans in Western culture? Since the spine is home to 800million nerve fibres, emerging through its various foramen—principally inbetween the spinal vertebrae—it is not an unreasonable assumption that much of the trouble begins here. Indeed, it is my experience as a physical therapist in various guises, for 25 years, that the spine is the principal source of all mechanical trouble. A brave claim you may say but one based purely on practice observation over thousands of patients. Certainly this is where I always begin my search for explanations even if the person arrives complaining of foot pains or pains in the top of the head or migraines!!
This will adequately justify on its own why the yogis who so ably developed the system we know, have made the entire study revolve around the spine. There is no posture that is not aimed at, in some way, improving the mobility of the spine— it is plain even on a superficial examination that all the readily taught postures in yoga classes have their principal effort aimed at improving the mobility of the whole spine. Thus we have several elements of spinal mobilisation which demonstrate that nerve trunks were aimed at. If we examine how the nerve roots emerge through the foramen formed by the upper and lower vertebrae at each

articulation of the spine, it is simple to see that there is great potential for disturbance to free movement of the spinal nerve root, either by way of intervertebral disc prolapse and subsequent compression of the nuclear contents upon the nerve trunk itself, or by what osteopaths call "irritability". This latter expression includes all those little parts of dysfunction that are described in this book and what we might label congestive processes. Immobility of an articulation means that there is a disturbance to the proper flow of fluids—blood and lymph principally but synovial exudates will also be affected. This may well have an effect upon the nerve trunk or root which is a living being, not like an electrical cable which only contains the live part with the plastic outer completely inert. The nerve coverings are requiring nutrition just like any other part and starvation will create reactions.

So the nerve trunks and roots all over have the potential to be compressed and if compression occurs there can be overt symptoms—tingling and numbness—but also covert symptoms. That is those which are below the consciousness of the individual—generally we would say that these are not at the moment threatening the person but can do in the future if there is no satisfactory resolution. It is most likely these sub-consciousness issues which readily resolve when taking up yoga, inducing so many people to claim that they feel more alive, better in themselves and any number of other descriptions which could not be justified on a purely technical basis.

The most threat to existence comes from compression of nerves as they emerge through the foramen. But there are also arteries, veins and lymph channels emerging through the same foramen. When one adds this fact then the prospects for serious interference become much more dramatic. Compressing a nerve root will have sufficiently bad long term consequences in themselves but if there is also compression of blood vessels and lymph channels then tissue life can be threatened. If blood does not reach a spinal structure say a ligament, in sufficient quantity, necrosis (tissue death) can occur or at least tissue starvation. The effects of this are poor regeneration and loss of elasticity along with the degenerative changes seen on post mortem examinations and to some extent on MRI scans. It is my belief that this is also the mechanism for degeneration of the hip joint and other cartilaginous areas but especially the spinal articulations.

If you choose to examine, especially, the books of dissection notes intended for medical doctors and trainee surgeons, you can quickly observe just how much material is contained within the human being, the proximity of so many different structures and just how much influence could be brought to bear by the action of compression.

There are other much less tangible aspects of the implications of malfunction for the nervous system. For example, if I as a practitioner were to test the average patient who attends with, say, a shoulder problem and test the strength of muscles surrounding the affected shoulder and then just do one very simple gentle neck stretch in one direction, it is frequently the case that the weak muscle just tested has returned to its normal strength. How can this be?? The same is the case for yoga-but it takes a little longer using only yoga. There is only one rational explanation----that the nerve compression/congestion and arterial/venous interference has been removed or reduced and the system is RETURNING TO NORMAL.

It is this feature of yoga which confuses so many—the system is not designed to make you something you have never been. I t works merely to replace you where you were –I consistently use the analogy of the child like state. Yoga will return you to how you were, perhaps even get you back to the state you enjoyed as a young person-not quite literally to the child state, of course!!

In much of the published material on anatomy and physiology there is no attempt made to explain the primary cause of degeneration. When the words arthritis and arthrosis are used it seems to be taken for granted that this is an inevitable process and accompanies ageing. Indeed, it has become identified with the ageing process, the two things being inextricably linked. It seems that few have bothered to examine why it does not occur in all humans—which it does not. Only the yogically oriented medics have bothered to discover that degeneration can be arrested in those taking up yoga, even when there were plainly visible physical signs of arthritic change, for example in finger joints. If degeneration can be arrested there has to be a good scientific reason!!

PART II. HOW YOGA SETS ABOUT SOLVING THESE PROBLEMS

At the end of this section, each posture will be analysed for its scientific effect upon the body. Where it is available, we will provide data that have been published in yoga scientific journals. These results will be from individual experiments carried out on people both who are adept at yoga and who have no knowledge but have been taught some yoga and have agreed to perform a certain range of posture over a set period of time— this time period has usually been 6 months which is considered sufficient time for changes to show their effects upon measurable processes such as blood pressure, digestion and so on. This will be from published data. What we say to the reader is that much of what is so far written in this book is the consequence of personal experience and observation in others—this, of course, is the principle upon which the complete yoga system is founded. Bear in mind that there were no dissections of bodies and no anatomy teaching establishments and no published works. All the knowledge came from within—also bear in mind that the origin of the word knowledge is the Greek GNOSIS –this means " to know from within"—it does not mean the acquisition of book learning which is the source of the vast majority of what people usually refer to as knowledge. The knowledge gained from within cannot be disputed and is not subject to ego because the person acquiring it does so gradually from his or her own personal practice. The body of inside knowledge comes routinely with effort applied in pursuit of truth so ego is not involved. The knowledgeable person has no axe to grind and no piece of paper to show for the gaining of this knowledge-he is content just understanding— perhaps this is a more appropriate word to use

1. General Analysis of How the Yoga System Works

The clue to how the system of yoga creates improvements is in the path taken by the body during adaptation - we generally use the term "getting stiffer"—in summary it is purely fascial shrinkage—and its movement towards the position of greater fascial length. If we are here contemplating just the physical benefits of yoga then it is easy to summarise the reason why it works as reversing those trends which so far have been imposed upon the body by the process of fascial adaptation— let us call this getting more flexible!. The most straightforward way of introducing this is by way of example. Ask our 5 year old to kneel with the left knee on the floor and the right leg extended out to the side. Then ask him to side bend over the right leg running the right hand down the right leg as far as possible. Ask this same person 30 years on to conduct the same test and there will be a considerable difference in the range attainable. This is so because of fascial shrinkage—adaptation to the habitual range of movement of the muscles around the waist. This has proved to be a most difficult concept to explain to the many thousands of patients and yoga students I and my colleagues have had over decades. Perhaps it would be more appropriate to state that it has been easy to EXPLAIN but difficult to understand by the vast majority of those to whom it has been explained. In reality it is no more difficult to comprehend than the notion of fecal elimination—unless one eliminates effectively then there will be health implications. Everyone takes this for granted, just as the cleaning of teeth is taken for granted. No-one has, in my experience, stated that tooth decay will be kept at bay by doing nothing. Any more than anyone would say that thirst or hunger are not natural indicators of the need to drink and eat. Yet---somehow it seems not possible for the vast majority to understand the notion of fascial adaptation. And then to go on to say this is so because it has not been prevented. Here, then, I propose to restate the obvious laws so that they may be put in proper context and be allowed to sit along side other very obvious laws which are taken for granted. I write these with tongue thrust gently into my cheek!!!!!-----

---Hunger will occur unless it is prevented—food is the cure
---Thirst will occur unless it is prevented—water is the cure
---Exhaustion will occur unless it is prevented—sleep is the cure
---Death will occur unless one breaths constantly.
---Death will occur if one jumps from a third floor window—not doing it will prevent death.

We could quite simply add many more what we could call obvious rules of living—and then right at the end add-----
--Fascia will shrink to adapt to the habitual range of use of the muscle unless it is prevented—stretching is the cure.

Placed within this simplistic list somehow it all seems to fit perfectly and be just as obvious-if you, the reader, see it thus, then my theory is probably correct—that one simply takes for granted all the other laws because they are so blindingly plain in every- day life and thus do not need stating. There is a further law and this is one that I like to compare with fascial shrinkage—the law of gravity. Again, no human being does not understand the law of gravity in its effects but few could accurately state it—all humans are expert in the manipulation of the law-the evidence for this is plain in every day life. Throw a ball of paper into your wastepaper basket—how did you know how much force to use? You demonstrated the need for a missile trajectory---you threw the ball upwards so that it would drop into the basket—the line drawn by the ball of paper is its trajectory and you demonstrated great expertise in the accurate throwing—even though it is likely that you have no idea as to the laws governing the trajectory!! For our understanding of yoga we need to take exactly the same attitude—except that in this book you will have a great deal more explanation of the laws governing the function of the human being than you would if you were studying gravity!!

Thus—the first and most important factor in the success of yoga postures is that the stretching of fascia takes place—and the effect of this is immediately to begin to undo the shortening that has taken place. Muscle fibres function most efficiently inside a fascial envelope that does not in any way constrain the fibres in their job of contracting and returning to full resting length—the product of antagonistic action. In other words the opposing muscle should then fully lengthen the other muscles. For an example take the bicep and tricep of the upper arm. If you straighten your arm, necessarily the bicep lengthens to its full length, If you fully flex your elbow then the tricep is fully lengthened—since this action takes place numerous times every day in the life of the average person, seldom does a bicep or tricep become contractured. (At this point it should be added that no muscles can lengthen itself—it must be lengthened by the action of the muscle opposite). And this daily repetition is the explanation for this. As a consequence, I have treated no more than 2 biceps or triceps in 25 years of practice---but thousands of hamstrings because no-one understands the need to perform the necessary forward bend every day to lengthen them. If school children were being taught by those who understand these simple natural laws, no doubt there would be a great deal less distress later in life.

How does the fascia stretch? The fascial envelope is much like a tough plastic bag—take hold of the bag and slowly place it under strong traction—it will plastically deform. But observe first-the bag is relaxed before you start. Then as you apply the traction you will sense a mild distortion of the material—hold this for a few seconds and then pull more strongly and hold this force. Then you will see that the plastic becomes longer and the lengthening remains after the force is removed. You can now say that the plastic has deformed permanently—this is known as plastic deformation whatever the material-it is even applied to steel. The human fascia behaves in an identical manner—except that it will shrink again unless the force is applied again. Now you may see that the rishis, the " seers " of thousands of years ago discovered this human characteristic, no doubt after realising that the child of 5 and the man of 50 did not compare in their movements. The man of 50 would have begun to stoop and shuffle perhaps—the rishis would then have taken some people and taught them the postures and seen that things could quickly be changed. Thus the system of yoga was born—and with millions of people having performed the posture over thousands of years, it has been refined until now, when it is possible to say that within the process of yoga there is nothing which does not work,; there is no unnecessary material; there is no technique which does not work; there is no confusing material. The process of refinement over thousands of years has provided a system which is **perfect**. However, there are circumstances that we encounter in our lives as therapists where we can speed up the process dramatically in order to render the patient pain- free much more quickly than would be the case just taking up yoga. It also is wise to recognise that the perfect system was designed for the Indian frame which is generally much slimmer than the Western frame and of course, has undertaken crossed-leg sitting and squatting since childhood.

The act of stretching plastically deforms the fascia making the plastic bag bigger and thus creating less compression upon its contents. This simple act sets off a chain of events which have monumental significance for humans—the body is beginning to go back to the state of childhood efficiency. The common retort is as follows........ "But surely you get stiffer as you get older?"—the reply is very simple....it is only so because you do nothing to prevent it. "But I play golf and go to the gym every week surely that should keep me supple?" No is the answer---go back to the first law which will be restated numerous times—shrinkage occurs unless you STRETCH and that takes time and can only be done SLOWLY holding the posture. No exercise enables this to occur. The ignorance of this simple fact is UNIVERSAL amongst therapists and orthopaedic specialists.

This improves the circulation and the quality of repair and maintenance of all tissues and thus counters the destructive effects of ageing. Muscles become more efficient because the blood and lymph flowing within moves with less resistance. In turn this means that effort can be reduced, because much energy has to be put into every day life just to overcome the effects of contractured muscle. The breathing systems create more efficient oxygen exchange reducing the rate of breathing. The heart rate and the blood pressure also decline. The person is able to sleep better and often for less time with less spinal stiffness. Digestion improves and elimination becomes more predictable and frequent. Organ and gland function improve because of the kneading and squeezing which occurs within the postures.

In summary-there is a whole health improvement. This is the amazing legacy which is yoga.

2. Genuine Stretching and its Effects

We are now going to take the issue of stretching and dissect it thoroughly so that you may understand the mechanisms at work. It is this aspect of yoga that is probably least understood—at many junctures there are comments made by those involved in yoga where the validity of postures being held static is questioned—it is this which made us realise that despite several thousand years of history there is still grave ignorance as to what is actually happening during a posture. Part of this difficulty emanates from the lack of trust in which intuition is held by modern people. It is a common teaching that knowledge comes from courses or books—that is, that knowledge comes from other sources than oneself. The Rishis discovered that humans have the capacity for the acquisition of deep understanding from introspective habits. The posture held for a couple of minutes provides the ground in which the aspirant can begin the journey of understanding why the posture makes him feel so much better. Any of the current group of new teachers coming from Shanti Yoga School would be able to tell you that their own yoga students in their beginners classes find that yoga is working for them. They tell this frequently to anyone listening even though these class participants have no idea why it is so!! This is the root of all real knowledge—the word knowledge emerges from the Greek word Gnosis which means to know from within. True knowledge is not facts learned parrot-fashion from books and teachers, but from self-study. How else could jalandhara banda have been discovered—how else could uddiyana banda have been discovered? These are physical characteristics that yogis discovered about the human body which no medically trained person has understood nor recognised.

We are, thus, considering why the act of true stretching works even though all those indulging in it do not know why they are doing it nor do they concern themselves with why it works. All they know –from within—is that it works. It works, in fact, for everyone who puts in the effort—it is not regulated by percentage; it is not restricted in whom it helps; it helps everyone who is willing to persevere. In the early 80's, I spent many weekends with people who lived with MS –all said that yoga helped them in so many ways even though none would say that they were " cured" by the practice of yoga.

In order to understand why and how it works it is essential to study the fascia since this is the material upon which the forces are acting. This is the material which the feeling of resistance and pain produce. The fascial system is not considered to be of any real relevance by the great majority of body work therapists. While it is recognised and alluded to there is only a handful of people accepting that it is the primary obstacle to full movement—of course yogis have the virtual monopoly since everything that is done in the way of postural work—work with asanas—is done in full recognition of the presence of fascial adaptation or shrinkage.

The system itself is vastly complex, an incredible mixture of relatively inelastic material, collagen, liquid lubricant, nerve endings and miles of fine blood vessels. In construction, we can take a crude parallel of a good quality wool jumper which has been washed in a washing machine on a programme that was too hot. The lovely new jumper is now a tight ball of wool. In the very simplest of terms this is what happens to fascia that is contractured. The word contracture is intended to convey the presence of hardening of muscle. Of course, to establish if a muscle is contractured it is necessary to FEEL it—something that is seldom done in any medical investigation. None of the thousands of patients I have treated has ever reported having their muscles palpated when facing a consultant or doctor—or ---I regret—a therapist-- of any kind. The word contracture appears in the medical literature but there are varying opinions as to how the word came about. We, of course, as fmm practitioners, recognise how to detect the presence of contracture since it is very obvious especially in the paraspinal muscles, trapezius, pectoralis major, rhomboids and a few others. Returning to our ball of wool—the fascial strands, which we refer to as a network of millions of strands-has become less lubricated, less mobile, there is now adherence of the fascial covering of the muscles to the bones it serves. This in itself squeezes the blood vessels and the nervous system reacts in the only way known to it-it creates pain. The mechanism by which pain is produced is either chemical—the build up of unexpelled products of metabolism (that is, toxins) or direct pressure on sensitive vessels. Or this could be both together. The contractured muscle necessarily restricts movement across the joints it covers and is capable of producing symptoms which can easily be identified as mimicking classic sciatic pain, for example.

When the muscle within its fascial envelope has its full mobility, there is no contracture. There cannot be pain from this muscle, at least not as a result of the processes described above.

Let us now contemplate the process of the reversal of this contracture and consider the mechanism of real stretching. Firstly, what should be understood is that the fascia has a tensile strength greater than steel. It behaves when forces of lengthening are applied, just as any other elastic material behaves. First it elastically deforms when force is applied. If this force is released then there is no plastic deformation-the material returns to its original contractured length. Now if a greater force of lengthening is applied, first the material will move through the elastic phase and then with continued holding of the stretching force, will begin to plastically deform. So we will now relate this to the act of performing a yoga posture. Let us say that you kneel on one knee and extend the other leg so that you end up in a gate posture. Now the arm nearest the bent knee is lifted overhead and the whole trunk is tilted sideways, moving into a side bend. The side that is opening up has three muscles with fascial layers—the internal and external oblique muscles which are overlaid by the transversalis, rather like a cummerbund as worn with a dinner jacket. These three layers of muscle are held at first in the "slack" attitude before the stretch is commenced. Thus phase one of the stretch is to take up the slack. Phase two comes with making a conscious attempt to persuade the trunk into side bending. Thus the second phase begins—the elastic phase. Then with more time holding and more effort applied the third phase is entered—the plastic deformation phase. This third phase causes much discomfort and necessitates much greater effort. After holding the stretch for at least 30 seconds—but more usually at least a minute—there will be actual lengthening of the fascial planes. Unless this third phase is entered there will be very little actual change in the fascial contracture. The ignorance of the need for this mechanism to be followed is almost universal within yoga circles since it has become almost fashionable to prevent yoga students from causing pain to themselves. Various strictures have been introduced into many UK training courses because—perhaps – of the fear of litigation. We know of a few people who are actively pursuing claims against yoga teachers, the students blaming the yoga teacher when in reality all yoga students must accept full responsibility for themselves. More of this later.

Now it can be understood, if you accept this concept, that plastic deformation-actual fascial lengthening—cannot take place unless there the three stages are employed. This dictates that postures must be held with strongly applied force. Thus this same characteristic cannot be achieved by any other means—certainly not be moving into and out of the posture without a static phase. What can be done by moving quickly is to create more heat which will soften the fascia and give the appearance of more flexibility-but this is delusional since softening declines to the norm when the activity ceases.

The concept of plastic deformation was fully documented in engineering. Hooke's Law was evolved just like Boyle's Law in physics, to show how metal deforms under stretching forces—and it behaves exactly as fascia because both are plastic in nature.

What actually happens during the full stretch almost requires no explanation when you consider the fascial contracture as if it were a ball of woolly jumper!! The blood vessels will be stretched making the flow of fluid much easier. The nerve endings will be moved apart and the muscle will be allowed to push out the products of metabolism thus relieving the congestive effect of inadequate movement. The fascial/periostial attachments of muscle to underlying bone which we refer to as adhesions, will quickly be changed as the joints are opened up. This will slacken the fascial bag in which the muscle is contained which in turn will promote the increased flow of blood. Lymph flow will improve. The nerve trunks which run in between the fascial clefts will have their compression relieved and will then be enabled to restore quality of nerve transmission as well as quality of nutrient supply to the nerve sheaths which are also living entities. In the case of spinal vertebral discs, the normal pumping mechanism which is grossly interfered with in the immobile position will be stimulated. In time the discs should at the very least be prevented from suffering further from excess unrelieved compression. Spinal veins and arteries which follow a tortuous route up the spine, will be continually and daily stretched thus not only improving the elasticity of the structures but easing congestion. The health of adjacent bone also will improve.

What has been described here is genuine stretching. Within our culture, and especially the culture of modern Western yoga, there is huge distortion as a result of deep fear. The common result is for only the first two parts of the three phase process to be undertaken—partly because there is inadequate time for the posture to be performed properly and partly because of lack of force. This word promotes a lot of fear—I make no apology for its use. On many occasions I have come up with alternatives such as "therapeutic discomfort "—but students of mine have seen through this disguise and laughed out loud at my attempt to disguise the truth. The truth is that one could not find a yogi who has transformed him or herself using yoga postures for whom the process was not painful. What is paramount in this process is that the student is comfortable with this notion—thus as a teacher I pass on this valuable piece of understanding, that one must move beyond the point at which there is any fear of the pain and do it regardless knowing that it will bring a great reward. When the reward arrives, the student can be seen smiling with understanding—it is this feature of the process of yoga that demands that the teacher act as guru, casting light on the dark and illuminating the students's path over sufficient time to enable this part of the journey to be undertaken without stopping to allow fear to prevent continuance. After that there is no longer any fear even though pain continues to be a feature of postural work for many years.

In a study of 5000people carried out by the New York and Columbia University –actually a random sample of back pain sufferers entering the hospital casualty departments, it was found that in 81% of the cases there was nothing more extraordinary than common or garden muscle spasm—muscle contracture of the erector spinae muscles in the lumbar spine. Another study was carried out independently by Dr Friedman of the ICD Rehab and Research Center, USA, and the very similar result was obtained.

This section of the book has been aimed at ensuring a basic but good understanding of what actually happens during a proper stretch since the word is used a lot in our culture and its meaning has been lost. Perhaps it would be more appropriate to write that we thoroughly explain the way we view a full stretch and this is not how it is normally viewed!

3. *Inversion*

Why not just hang upside down from a tree by your ankles?—this question has been put to me on several occasions, particularly when in conversation with those who wish to consider that a piece of equipment like a back swing could produce just the same results as a headstand. Since yoga has been refined in the crucible of time for thousands of years the humble will permit the notion of historical value to over-ride any consideration of superior knowledge. But let us look at the process of inverted posture and see why inversion is so valuable.

Since the head stand has been called rajasana—king of postures—this must be the place to begin our analysis. We can commence with published results of scientifically devised trials conducted by medical, Western trained doctors. Drs. Bhole and Chandra are notable amongst the experimenters whose work has been published in recognised medical journals

The flow of blood within the brain-not the whole head—does not increase despite popular mythology. What does occur is that those arteries which are poorly served with blood receive a signal via their baroreceptors—pressure receivers—to open up, to dilate. Those arteries that are well served close down via the same mechanism. There is thus, a redistribution of blood rather than an increase. It is this factor which is linked by scientists to the improvements to concentration and memory which ensue from regular head stand performance.

The head stand drains about half a litre of blood from the legs over a period of about 5 minutes, which ends up around the throat, neck muscles and forearm muscles thus engorging the thyroid with blood and improving its ability to function. There is an increase in the consumption of calories during the posture despite the heart rate declining—this is the only exercise known to man which exhibits this characteristic.

Experiments have shown that there is a 50% increase in oxygen over the standing position whilst slowing the heart rate by 10-15 beats per minute. There is considered to be an improvement in the pattern of blood flow within the brain and it seems that it is unlikely that any increase in blood pressure during the posture will result in damage to tissue because of the increase in blood flow and pressure within the forearm which acts as a sort of sink for the redistributed blood. Sometimes this has been called the slimmers posture!!

There is quite obviously strong compression upon the neck vertebrae. This will cause the intervertebral discs to be squeezed hard thus stimulating the nocturnal imbibition characteristic. This feature of human biology goes wrong on so many people—it may have been understood thousands of years ago—if this is so(-we speculate that it is so--), then it may help to explain why yogis have not been suspended by their ankles-we believe that it is essential for compression to take place. Clearly, in this attitude there is no compression. It can also be demonstrated that the act of performing something like the plough followed by the cobra will have a far more profound effect upon the joint surfaces then suspension could offer.I have taken a tape measure and assessed the length of the spine at the front and back in both these two postures, and in suspension, and there is far more lengthening in the postures than in suspension.

Experiments by A. Bouhys, the results of which were published in the Journal of Applied Physics, found that in people tilted passively from the upright position to the upside down position did not manifest the same phenomena as displayed during the headstand, with the exception of the excursion of abdominal contents.

During the headstand the walls of the leg veins collapse and when the surfaces come into contact with one another, there is a release of thrombin, an anti-coagulant, an anti-blood clotting agent.

The abdominal contents gradually will move downwards until they rest upon the diaphragm—this can be felt by the adept. This naturally relieves pelvic congestion which is an important source of abdominal problems. The weight of the abdominal contents will therefore rest upon the liver and transverse colon thus compressing them. Alternate compression and decompression are the primary source of maintenance of efficient function of abdominal organs. The brain blood distribution has been mapped by sending a radio-active isotope through the blood stream.

Now let us further consider the neck vertebrae. The act of compression upon the vertebrae—the amount of force for the average person is around 11 stone, moving from about 10 pounds from pure head weight----- is augmented by the process of venous drainage. The tortuous route taken by the vertebral veins and arteries through the neck, makes it a strong likelihood that blood flow will be restricted in the human being, this is despite youth and vigour. The animal usually has its head down so is unlikely to suffer from this. The animal neck, if it is continually in the head down position, is constantly subjected to traction—lengthening—so will not see the effects of blood flow restrictions for the same reasons as the human being. The head will also often come up above the heart— thus for the animal the head down-head up position is regular during a normal day. For the adult Westerner, it is very unlikely that inversion will ever take place unless there is a yoga routine. We could speculate that when adults decide to not permit the head down position on the grounds of dizziness or some other perceived undesirable characteristic, there is then a deterioration of the systems which are naturally in place to prevent such aberrations taking place. A sort of biological Catch 22??

The maintenance of continuous compression on spinal vertebral articulations creates immobility, even just because of the load. That is so even before considering the impact of the failure to actually MOVE them! So any relief must benefit the processes which work continuously to move in repair materials and to discard waste products.

The fears and anxieties of performing this posture, these being more regularly propounded in yoga circles than ever before, are based upon the what I call " one foot in the grave concept"—most people would recognise Murphys Law perhaps!! Or Sods Law.

This really means that if something could possibly go wrong then it most probably will. It is a most easily understood concept—provided you have the "one foot in the grave" mind –set. Yoga tends to attract largely positive people so it is more curious that so many should allow themselves to be persuaded of the dangers of anything before considering the massive benefits. We could take the car as a prime example. If I say to you that every year in UK there are 4000 deaths in RTA's and there are

170,000 serious injuries in vehicles and there are 400,000 vehicles written off each year—how does driving to work feel now?? The home creates more accidents than any other place—far more than motoring accidents-how does that feel? So it is a great surprise to continually hear of prohibitions on the performance of the headstand. Take me to someone who has been injured performing the headstand—give me the name of someone who you personally know has suffered after performing the headstand. The risk is miniscule and it is a risk that can easily be analysed—if you are likely to fall then simply practise in the corner of a room where falling is not possible. There is a risk inherent in EVERYTHING we do as humans—life is hazardous wherever you look—so why pick that posture that has been named the King of Postures?? Even when I put this logic to some class participants they refuse to make the attempt. When those who are fearful do persevere and master the headstand they emerge as having a profoundly different attitude!

What becomes apparent to those involved in yoga is that the negative messages transmitted by some emanate from two primary sources. Firstly those outside yoga—physios, osteopaths, chiropractors—so called experts who have never practised yoga but proclaim some special knowledge and thus hoodwink the unthinking—and then there are those within, pre-eminent amongst which is one particular organisation which claims to speak for the whole of the yoga world. Listening to some of the teachers who have trained at the BWY it is small wonder that there are prohibitions imposed—the teacher creates fear and does not master the fear and then passes this fear on to students who know no better. This I have discovered amongst many BWY teachers over many years—I have not encountered one who could give a good analysis of the hazards of any posture—but many were acclaimed antagonists. Of course, what usually transpired during discussions was that their own teachers had passed on THEIR fears and these had never been put under the microscope. Part of the purpose of this book is to subject all postures to analysis so that some of these absurdities can be eliminated. However—there is another realisation that goes with the territory described—most people who are in fear have fears that are so deep rooted that only the strongest of efforts—fortitude, perseverance etc—could shift them. Yoga, then, is not the issue—the issue is fear of living!!

Inversion is a deeply established part of yoga - is it conceivable that the yogis of thousands of years ago got it badly wrong?? In my view—NO.

The common retort I receive when going through this analysis is this___"Ah yes, that is all very well but would you persuade a 60 year old with spondylitis to go straight into the headstand?" You may see that it is a common human characteristic to pick out the extraordinary rather than the average!

4. Compression

With consideration, one can begin to see that what happens in yoga is that there is constant compression, decompression, shearing, twisting, inversion, pulling---and so on. There is, thus, an attempt to produce the notion of constant motion. This does not mean that there is never any rest nor any stopping but if you examine the average day, there are few occasions of total immobility. Probably the computer and the modern car are the direct cause of most of the modern immobility!!

Compression is created by gravity throughout life for all living things. Most mammals sleep lying down, thus removing spinal compression. However, the effect of just lying down is very small —consider the lengthening of the spine as the gauge. If you measure your spine on rising you would find that you are about 1-2 inches taller than at the end of the day. This is entirely attributable to disc rehydration—the spinal discs have filled up with fluid. The compression placed upon them on rising will effectively squeeze out the new fluid and the process will begin again the next day—providing the vertebrae are not immobile. Now if you measure the length of the spine during the forward bend it is more like 4 inches longer-but, obviously, only at the rear. Then if you perform the cobra or camel and measure the front of the spine, it will be found that there is a similar amount of lengthening. This amount cannot be reproduced by hanging upside down, nor by traction—the amount when performing the postures is greater. This is because the FASCIA is actively stretched. — traction does not have enough power to do this—although if you were to put a body on an old fashioned torture rack, the fascia would certainly be lengthened!! But no-one will do this!! In the forward bend, naturally, there is also muscular effort and the **will** is strengthened. Obviously these are absent in torture!

The compression is both abdominal and structural. The abdominal contents are heavily compressed during certain postures, increasing the blood flow enormously. The compressive force is what obstructs blood flow and the release of the compressive effort and subsequent stretching in an opposing posture permits a greater tidal flow of fluids.

Compression on cartilage pumps it up. Walking will permit the hip and knee cartilage to thicken and toughen, preparing this for more arduous tasks such as running.

The compression upon intervertebral discs is probably the most significant feature of yoga postures from the perspective of long term spinal health. It is my view that long term integrity of the spine is heavily dependent upon the strength of discs. In all manuals of physical assessment the discs are usually referred to as wearing away with age. The expression used is "dehydration". In other words, age makes them dry out and –so the notion goes—this will predispose the owner to less troublesome back pain. However, most of the books have been written by those who know nothing of yoga and who have only knowledge of ill people-hospital cases. It is a fair guess that the spines of yogis have not been MRI scanned to find out the disc hydration signal strength.

So—compression regularly applied to the human spine we believe has a profound affect upon the integrity of discs. There have been numerous studies performed on yogis and non-yogis in Indian yoga hospitals to establish what happens with spondylitis and spondylosis of the neck. These studies have been x-ray studies so actually only bony characteristics are seen but the tests have conclusively shown that bony deterioration of vertebrae has been halted and sometimes reversed by the performance of yoga postures. Compressive postures such as the shoulder stand and head stand have been part of the programme even when the person has serious degeneration of neck vertebrae.

Compression on the skull during the headstand has no beneficial effect as far as we understand it—it always hurts even after 20 years—but since the bones of the skull are reputed to be mobile it may well be that, just as cranial osteopathy manipulates these ones, so may this posture. We can offer a further speculation that the weight increase upon the skull and the huge increase in the forces applied to blood within the head will have a beneficial effect upon the movement of cerebrospinal fluid, especially as recent research has shown that the previously considered fascial make-up being solid material has now been shown to be tubular and filled with – CS fluid!

5. Decompression

It has been demonstrated that the alternate compression and decompression is what maintains the health of tissues such as cartilage. It has also been shown during tests on yoga students that the **constant** state of compression OR decompression will produce degeneration. It therefore must be concluded that it is the act of **variation** that produces the benefit. This benefit must be bestowed because there is constant alternation. It is simple to find this characteristic for yourself. If you stand in bare feet and not moving soon your feet will begin to hurt—they will ache. If you begin to walk as soon as this aching is apparent, it is only minutes until the ache has disappeared. The message is plain—standing still will begin to overstretch foot ligaments and it is this characteristic which will create the aching. Nature is sending you a message—don't stand immobile—move around and alternate between standing and sitting. This may provide a clue as to why most poor people have always adopted the cross-legged sitting posture—it does not create this characteristic since we have acquired two sitting bones, called in technical language, the ischial tuberosities. These are well enough padded for most people not to be bothered by aching since there are no ligaments involved to become overstretched.

In all the strong postures there will be alternate compression and decompression. The actual act of compression and its relief, is mostly of benefit to those structures such as organs and cartilage but we must not neglect the fact that in order to produce the act of compression and its counterpart there must be strong muscular effort which itself has great and obvious benefits.

Bones become brittle and porous and weakened not because of age but because of lack of use. Bone is not a shock absorber—the absorption of shock is the job of muscle and fascia. But the loading of bones is vital for their health so that compression-and decompression- of bone is the principle component of this process. Yoga provides the way for all people regardless of age to maintain the integrity of bone by the application of load gradually applied. The argument in the West has often been to advise against exercise for such conditions as hip joint deterioration but this is based upon false premises. Whilst the degenerating hip joint will be painful and therefore should not be subjected to unnecessary loading, the rest of the body will deteriorate unless load is applied. In this regard yoga cannot be surpassed. For the person with a seriously deteriorating hip joint it would be best to avoid such things as jogging or running because of the effect upon cartilage.

We can at this juncture consider the act of decompression of the spinal vertebrae to be VITAL for the health of the spine----this must surely be one of the main components to justify sleeping lying down since it is only the act of attaining the horizontal position that enables the spinal intervertebral discs to decompress—and it is this which enables them to fill with new liquid to replace the old. This constant daily routine of spinal compression and decompression is what maintains the integrity of the discs and the loss of decompression opportunity is the primary reason for disc ruptures. This loss of opportunity occurs because myofascial structures surrounding the spine have become contractured and thus do not permit expansion. The effect of shortened myofascial structures is the constant tourniquet. This incredibly simple concept is not understood in any branch of medicine even though extensive experiments have been conducted to ascertain the nature of nocturnal imbibition --all these conducted by surgeons and investigators within the established medical system—here we see a wonderful example of how what would be called knowledge has not even been used to help patients having spinal surgery to understand why the disc has burst. Surgeons simply do not tell the patients why they have incurred this problem and what cold be done to prevent a recurrence. Here we can see another example of what I refer to as Internet Knowledge. Lots of patients now come armed with material published on the internet which is useless for most intents and purposes primarily because it has been published by people who just do not UNDERSTAND the significance of what has been written—it is just written down to acquire some piece of paper or to pass an examination or to impress colleagues. It does not contribute to a change of procedure when dealing with patients with spinal trouble –this is most apparent at GP level where the " pills and rest "formula for the bad back is alive and going strong –and, unfortunately, the term " slipped disc" is still common currency!

6. Joint Mobilisation

If there is one feature—of course this is not possible—that we had to choose this would be it. In our work as therapists we see spinal joint immobility every day of our therapy working lives. Yoga has more to offer than any other process.

Let us consider the construction of a typical spinal joint. The word joint is our first problem—the juxtaposition of vertebrae are technically speaking not the true joint. The vertebrae and disc attached and the next vertebrae are better referred to as a unit of articulation. They certainly do articulate with one another but not in the same manner as, for example, the knee joint. In this joint the rolling surfaces are lubricated by synovial fluid excreted by the capsule surrounding the joint. The stimulus to excrete is produced by movement. The spinal vertebrae have no capsule nor is the disc innervated—it has no nerves. Neither is there any blood supply to the disc—the nutrient is entirely dependent upon compression and decompression –and naturally the quality of ingested nutrient strongly influences the quality of fluid pumped into the disc.

Aside from the absence of a capsule and nerves and blood supply then we have a similar problem in the spinal articulations to that faced by synovial joints. The demand is that they are kept mobile. Actually, the Full Movement Method of physical therapy has been distilled from yoga to achieve precisely this. It is our experience that the restoration of the full range of movement to spinal joints causes a removal of pain. We have, thus, concluded that every joint must be moved through its full range in order to prevent any symptoms. The presence of symptoms is, in our minds, entirely the result of a loss of range. The loss has to be quite substantial before symptoms appear, however, but nevertheless when they do appear they can quickly and easily be removed by applying processes which restore the range.

We do not claim that this is original thinking –indeed it has been known in physiotherapy for decades. What we claim is that whilst it is known it is not practised nor when it is practised by a few, is it done with yogic understanding. Joint mobilisation is often "wrench and hope" –this is the feature of chiropractic we least believe in whereas fmm actually mimics yoga postures and thus produces no distress in the patient nor any tearing of tissue.

The common construction of vertebral articulations of the bod
have ligaments binding the periosteums together—the periosteur.
covering of each bone—with tiny muscles attaching each vertebrae to
those above and below. These muscles are referred to as the rotators—
meaning that they aid in rotating the bone against its neighbour. These
"rotatores" are fascially bound as are all muscles. In the case of vertebrae
there are also what are often referred to as facet joints—the proper name
is apophyseal—these are genuine synovial joints and also have fascial
bindings. Each vertebra, because a plentiful supply of blood is required to
all the structures surrounding each bone, as well as the bone itself, has
numerous veins and arteries and these take a tortuous route along the
length of the spine. Any straightening out of this pipework system creates
improvements in flow.

Now we can examine the process of joint mobilisation with a grasp of
what structures are likely to be affected by any mobilisation effort we
make. This is the sole purpose of section 13 of the book—an analysis of
what actually happens in each posture.

Moving from spinal articulations to major joints let us consider what one
very famous yogi—a medical doctor as well as a practising yogi—had so
say about joints;

"The joint cavity is lined with delicate synovial membrane which secretes
synovial fluid to lubricate the joint. The cells of the joint depend on a
fairly tenuous blood supply for their vital requirements. If the circulation
of prana in a joint is blocked or deficient over a long period of time, the
supply of blood and lymphatic fluid becomes sluggish and the joint fluid
grows stagnant. When this occurs the waste products and poisons of
cellular metabolism build up in the lubricating fluid of the joint, rather
than being efficiently transported to the skin and kidneys for elimination
from the body. Acidic wastes and toxins, accumulating in the joint fluid,
irritate the sensitive nerve fibres in the joint causing pain and stiffness. If
the circulation of fluid and prana remains interrupted for a long time, the
structure of the joint itself begins to dry up and the soft cartilage lining
corrodes. The bones then begin to accumulate excessive calcium, forming
new bone growth which limits movement."
Bhole, Dr. M.V., M.D. 1973, Deputy Director of Scientific Research at
Kaivalyadhama Research Institute in occasional research papers entitled:
"Some Physical Considerations of the Asanas".

It would be hard to improve on that succinct definition.

7. Diaphragm and Heart Function

Examining the dissection notes of surgeons it is easy to see that the heart is fascially bound to the diaphragm. So is the liver. If you were setting off to design the human body and you did not intend for the heart to be affected by the diaphragm I suggest that it would have been easy to glue it to the sternum—by which it is, in any event, partially protected from direct blows. If as a designer you were not sure what to do perhaps you could just have left it to hang beneath the lungs, but sitting on top of the diaphragm. A pump will work anywhere—take a pond pump as an example—just suspend it or stick it on the bottom of the pond and it will function just as well regardless of its position. The same is true of the human body-the heart could go anywhere. But the creator has made a conscious decision—it is so heavily bound to the diaphragm that separation would only be possible by scalpel. It is clearly intended to remain there and to be influenced by the movement. The same can be said of the liver—whilst most people learning anatomy and physiology would know that the liver is massaged by the diaphragm, few would recognise that the heart's attachment has a far greater and deeper significance. It is not bound to the diaphragm to keep if from moving about-the tie is not to immobilise it—the reason for the heart being fascially tied to the diaphragm is to ensure that it receives constant mobilisation. Why is this necessary? I believe that this is organised in this manner entirely because the fascial covering—the pericardium-will shrink just like all other fascia unless it is stretched. And the only way in which this can be achieved is to attach it to that which creates relative movement more than any other structure. It has also to be recognised that the heart is fascially tied to the neck and to the sternum. –this simple device ensures that some yoga postures will be supremely effective in stretching the whole heart! At this point is may be instructive to extract a part from one of the surgeons dissection books that medical students use—even this clearly states the purpose of this attachment

"The positions given are only approximate because the heart is a mobile organ whose shape and position varies with diaphragmatic movement and venous return. Thus if a deep breath is taken and expiration attempted against a closed mouth and nose, the heart is narrowed by a reduction in venous return caused by the high intrathoracic pressure and elongated by the lowering of the diaphragm. The converse effect is produced by attempting to inspire against a closed nose and mouth after full expiration."

A further interesting section appears adjacent in the same dissection notes.

"The diaphragmatic surface of the heart is formed entirely to accommodate the ventricles of the heart and this is referred to as a sulcus (an indentation). The sulcus contains the posterior interventricular branch of the right coronary artery and the middle cardiac vein." There is a picture of the underside of the heart—what is referred to as its diaphragmatic surface—which shows all the blood vessels. There is a right coronary artery, having two major branches, there is the circumflex branch of the left coronary artery with its several branches and the beginning of the great cardiac artery along with the great cardiac vein and several of its branches. All these vessels pass under the diaphragmatic surface of the heart and are contained within the overall pericardiac sheath and are, of course, subject to compression from the weight of the heart and the upward force created by the diaphragm itself, this compression only relieved when the diaphragm is brought downwards by the deep breath. Again, it has to be accepted that this is a logical conclusion. In this particular series of surgeons dissection notes, the more of it is read the more it is apparent that even an anatomist has seen the reality of the design!!!!
Romanes, G. J. Professor. CBE., Ph.D., FRCS. *Manual of Practical Anatomy* Vol.2, Oxford University Press .Ed 14.)

"Blood vessels , aorta and vena cava pass through that part of the diaphragm where less action takes place. Arcuate ligaments protect the aorta from ever being affected by the action of the diaphragm and vena cava ONLY in deep breathing when the diaphragm aids return of blood to the heart."
Todd, M.E. 1937+59 *The Thinking Body*
Princeton Book Company, New Jersey USA.

"The inferior vena cava pierces and fuses with the central tendon of the diaphragm 2-3cm to the right of the median plane. When the diaphragm contracts it compresses the abdominal viscera, lowers the intrathoracic pressure and pulls the inferior cava open, thus facilitating the flow of blood from the abdomen into the thorax". (**Romanes, G. J.** Professor. CBE., Ph.D., FRCS. *Manual of Practical Anatomy* Vol.2, Oxford University Press .Ed 14.) This could not be anymore explicit—the diaphragm is attached and is necessarily attached. It is done on purpose. But even this dissector may not have seen what is the effect of this opening of the pipe—its distension. The act of distension must be followed by a narrowing and this sudden change makes the action into a pumping action—thus the diaphragm is a second heart. Unlike the actual heart, of course, it is easily prevented from doing its work by too much immobility. It is also possible by experiment to determine from palpating oneself that in the act of running and forced rapid breathing, such as is inevitable with runners generally, that the diaphragm does not move as it does when performing a yoga posture. Since the runner subjects her body to forces at the foot which are three times body weight, it is again a reasonable assumption that the blood in the legs –especially- is impeded not just because of this gravitational effect but because only one of the pumps is working correctly. The return pump—the diaphragm—is impeded in its function because of the speed it is required to work at during running. I am sure that if one were able to scan the diaphragm during running its excursion would be minimal. Bear in mind that blood flow for the runner should be maximal. Surely with this knowledge it can be deduced that blood flow may actually be minimal and thus the heart has to do not only the supply function but the return function as well. It could explain why runners hearts are often seen to enlarge pathologically and them to die younger than their supposed level of fitness would imply was likely. The yogis, of course, stated that heavy physical exercise was destructive!

A recent discovery in another publication which has been in my library for 25 years and which has never been read from cover to cover, is as follows;

"From Postural Balance and Imbalance, the American Academy of Osteopathy------ (American Academy of Osteopathy, 1975. Occasional Papers presented at the Academy and published under the title; *Postural Balance and Imbalance.* **Peterson, B** (Ed.))

As has been pointed out the flow of venous blood depends to a great extent upon the normal muscular activity and fascial tension. The large veins of the abdomen pass through and are attached to the diaphragm, the motion of which is of great importance in moving the blood within the veins. Restricting the diaphragmatic function is then capable of increasing the chronic passive congestion of all the venous channels below this level."

This is the most deliberate and direct reference to diaphragmatic control of venous flow that I have ever read and goes far beyond any anatomical statement, aligning itself fairly and squarely with my own conclusions based upon research and observation and profound internal assessment. I have begun to alert yoga students to this phenomenon especially those who are new to teaching. I have used a variety of suggestions for establishing the truth of this, one of which is to force breath holding and feel the increase in pelvic congestion as a result.

It may be worth stating –again quoting the surgeons notes, that two neck vertebrae give nerve branches to the phrenic nerve which serves the diaphragm—in fact from the C3 to C5 including the fourth. Inherent in this design is plenty of potential of interference from neck malfunction, maybe indirectly affecting the diaphragm. This is hard to prove. Lots of patients with neck problems report immediate improvements in breathing following neck treatment.

.It is my view that this explains the presence of angina pains for many people—this view has some substance especially when you see that angina is quickly cleared or "cured" when a person takes up yoga. However, I stress that this is a logical deduction from what is apparent— but this does not guarantee that it is a fact. The yogis of yore have stated that exercise is unnecessary for the maintenance of circulatory health— most commonly known as cardiovascular health. By this term is meant the pipework and the heart as well as the lungs. Here it would be valuable to provide a synopsis of the findings of a particular cardiac surgeon who goes against the whole culture by saying that the evidence for hard physical exercise being helpful in prolonging life and health is WRONG!! His series of statements runs counter to all that popular writing has taken as Gospel truth-and he refutes all current stereotypes by producing lots of EVIDENCE. Here is a summary of his findings—which I have to say are as hard-hitting as the others presented in this book from my own experience!

"Fitness and health are distinct and independent of one another.

"Cardiovascular health refers to the absence of disease and implies nothing about the actual health of your arteries or your heart."

"Coronary heart disease can be silent and produce no symptoms"

"But there is no evidence that a slower resting heart rate is healthier than a heart rate somewhat faster or that a quicker return to resting heart rate after exercise is inherently beneficial. There are people who have proven rapid heart rate who are in their eighties and apparently have good health."

"As for increasing maximum oxygen consumption when you are exercising at your peak, there is certainly nothing intrinsically healthier about that. Athletes frequently have abnormal electrocardiograms, manifesting changes that in non-athletes would be considered unmistakeable signs of heart disease."

"The most common purpose of stress testing is to find out whether you do or don't have coronary heart disease. That's what the Committee on Exercise of the American Heart Association says and that is what most doctors think they are doing when they suggest you take a stress test. Implied in this notion is that if the stress test does not reveal coronary heart disease then you can conclude with confidence that you are free from it. The trouble is that this conclusion is wrong. You can have a test which shows that you do not have a good work capacity but your heart arteries are perfect and you can have furred up arteries but pass the stress test."

Let us finish with this---from the same source

"Some assume that when they are enrolled in a planned prescribed or supervised exercise program they can safely abdicate responsibility for their own safety. They feel they need not worry about overdoing it because the plan has been chosen by an expert. Others, no matter how expert they are, cannot know how much, how far and for how long you should exercise on any given day. Fitness is not related to health at all. Heart attacks are not prevented by exercise. Exercise may provoke heart attacks. The exercise fad is a folly and a danger. It only takes you to spread the word."

This is a little book with a big message—interestingly the author comes up with walking as the best exercise-not quite enlightened enough to realise yoga might do the job even better. The source is Dr Henry Solomon writing in his little book "The Exercise Myth". (Solomon, Dr.H. MD. *The Exercise Myth*. F.A.Davis Company Philadelphia, USA 1981.)

What has been stated by yogic scientists after extensive tests is that in virtually all comparisons of control groups with people doing yoga postures and those performing the Canadian Air Force 5BX programme of exercises, yoga emerges as more effective than any other mechanism for improving overall health. This is the case even for muscle strength tests –we believe that this is the case not because of any inherently superior model of muscle working but because of the removal of inhibiting influences. The major researchers into yoga are clear in their assertion that no increase in muscle bulk will take place with yoga.

It is this action which should be sufficient to convince even the most ardent sceptic that we have two hearts—only one, however, is recognized as significant in the passage of blood.

In general we can see that the action of yoga postures will have a more profound effect upon the fascia –the pericardium—than any exercise and it may be that this is why the author of the book earlier referred to has gathered his conclusions. He has come to similar conclusions as have we but for slightly different reasons. In fact, it could easily be that the marathon runner who gets such a bad press in Dr Solomons book, strains his heart because the fascia is too tight and that the diaphragm does not function efficiently when the breathing is so rapid as it must be during fast running. We will examine in considerable detail the workings of these two major structures when we contemplate the individual yoga postures. (Solomon, Dr.H. MD. *The Exercise Myth*. F.A.Davis Company Philadelphia, USA 1981.)

Now we may consider the diaphragm itself. This structure is referred to, regularly in anatomy and physiology books, as "the flat sheet of muscle which separates the abdominal cavity from the thorax."

Whilst its purpose is recognised, it value is not. What can be seen in people even of teenage years, is its failure to function in the manner for which it as designed. We can see this quite easily if examining a teenage boy. Look at him, unclad on the torso, from a side view. Even with absolutely no knowledge of posture you will be able to see the flat chest, rounded shoulders. Many parents who bring their children for treatment, plead with me to "tell them its bad for them". It is an unfortunate fact that at 14 it is almost too late and the saying "too little, too late," springs immediately to mind. Unless the boy is suddenly about to dedicate himself to considerable change then things will stay much as they are now, at the very best. So -----what has happened since the age of 5, to turn this upright body into a stooping incipient old person? Principally, he has sat too much and sat hunched over a machine; the first noticeable characteristic would have been hamstring shortening and this would have been obvious around age 5 but far more apparent at age 9 after 4 years of school. It is the sitting and the compressive effect upon the hamstring structures which have caused the muscle fascia to shrink far more than at any point in the child's body. This is easily verifiable—if you observe the infants at age 5 and then trace the same youngsters at the junior school level and then—especially the boys—see these same people at the senior school, you will be given a lesson in body mechanics. There will be a movement of the head and neck of the 5 year old—the head will be straight on top of the perfectly upright neck – forward just enough in the 9 year old for you to observe the movement from the vertical to the slightly inclined. This will increase in the senior school, bringing more inclination to the neck but far more importantly, there will be a depression of the rib cage for the vast majority of boys. Girls appear to be less affected-I have not worked out why this is so but it certainly can be observed. It may be that boys are more inclined to work on personal electronic machines and are thus bent forward more but there is another more sinister possibility—that they are actually depressed. In 2005, the medical profession reported that 160,000 prescriptions for anti-depressants were given to under-16's---. What I do not know is the gender split.

What does the depressed posture do? It shrinks the fascia around the abdominal muscles which as they progressively shorten, will pull down the rib cage, reducing the volume of air available for oxygen exchange. Whilst it is my belief that the human body is sufficiently intelligent to make do even when this is extreme, it is certain that the diaphragm quality of function is severely compromised and this will have radical consequences for abdominal organ health because of deprivation of muscular massage to the contents of the abdomen. This massage affects the heart, blood flow, liver and small and large intestine though the active youngster will not notice any loss because youth will protect him. More serious abdominal consequences will occur in later life. Certainly GP's report massive amounts of constipation which are stated as being the result of immobility.

The fascial shrinkage creates a difficulty for the diaphragm to function correctly. The connections from the diaphragm to the base of the ribs are there to enable the sheet of muscle to be flattened as well as drawn down—the twin action is important for full function and to engage the full effect of the diaphragmatic contraction. This is, as has been shown in earlier chapters, the main provider of return blood flow to the heart. So it could be speculated that the combined effect of immobility, which is the modern work pattern, and the loss of diaphragmatic function will cause the heart to be under constant compression which itself will be unrelieved for long periods. It should be plain that the antidote is the cobra posture or the camel and this will be thoroughly examined in the relevant postural sections

The movement of the ribs outwards during a strong in-breath, is what creates the stimulus for the vena cava to be opened and closed, acting as a heart.

In the slumped posture this function will be considerably curtailed perhaps halted altogether. Unless the owner of the body is made aware of this function then they will remain in ignorance of the true value of the diaphragm. It should be said, however, that all those young people that I have told have not done anything to change the situation –so one could easily become quite cynical about humanity.

The diaphragm is the structure which draws in air to the lungs. The person whose diaphragm does not function properly—or at least it is not being used-can be seen to be breathing clavicularly. This is indicated by the rise and fall of the collar bones during breathing and is typical of asthmatics and bronchitics. The diaphragm sucking air down into the lungs is important if the lung tissue is to be used in its intended manner—rather as a jug is filled from the bottom up should lungs be so filled in this way.

This is a major part of the value of yoga breathing exercises. Over 20 years of teaching yoga and even more treating human bodies has shown me that there are, even amongst the fit and healthy, at least 50% of people whose diaphragm does not function in the prescribed manner and needs stimulating until it works properly.

To gauge this, it is a simple matter for you to put your hands around the base of your ribs—in a manner similar to putting your hands on your hips—and press inwards and then attempt to make a full breath against your own hand -applied resistance. Unless you can feel your ribs giving a very strong force to overcome your hand strength then poor function is demonstrated. In the example of the young person having poor posture, the more significant feature is the loss of fascial mobility. This imposes an actual physical blockage to proper function, strapping the ribs down so firmly that sideways movement will be interfered with. This physical restriction is in addition to the loss of innate ability which would have been present at the age of 5. It is this loss of innate ability—by definition it is not realised since it is unconscious—that prevents the person from understanding that there has been a loss. This may well explain why so many people become sick with serious diseases without knowing that something is going wrong until the disease is well under way.

Worry immobilises the diaphragm because worry affects the solar plexus—the seat of "butterflies" which itself is a manifestation of solar plexus nerve interference—and worry is cited by many authorities as the primary cause of cancer. Actually FEAR would be a more appropriate word.

8. Brain

At the VHS Medical Centre in Madras, India numerous experiments have been conducted into the effects of yoga. These have all been carefully controlled trials performed upon subjects who were not previously conversant with yoga and had agreed to perform a series of postures as part of an experiment to discover if yoga works more effectively than drugs in controlling certain diseases.

The introduction to these experiments is done by stating that many mental and bodily diseases are caused by stresses of normal every day life. In susceptible individuals stress can produce psychomatic illnesses like high blood pressure, bronchial asthma, thyrotoxicosis, peptic ulcer, and may also precipitate such psychiatric disorders as schizophrenia, epilepsy, aggression and drug addiction.

At the Medical centre, chemicals were measured before and after 6-9 months of yoga practice. These chemicals were metabolites of biogenic amines and adrenal cortical hormones and also EEG recordings of psychiatric patients' disorders. There was considerable improvement in the condition of the patients after yoga therapy with restoration of normal levels of biogenic amines.

Diabetics with a fasting level blood sugar above 150mg were chosen for part of the study. Severe cases of bronchial asthma not responding to medical treatment were chosen. Patients with hypertension consisting of systolic pressure of above 170mg and diastolic above 100mg were chosen. There were 20 patients in each of 6 groups listed as above. All patients were given yoga asanas mostly of the type practised in any yoga class in the West. The asthmatics were also taught pranayama and meditation was taught to the aggressive and epileptic patients.

The theory was that these various ailments were the result of disturbances in the balance of chemicals in the blood and those chemical substances produced in the brain—the neurotransmitters. These medical scientists have found evidence before that upsets in these balances create substantial behavioural changes. Examples of neurotransmitters are noradrenaline, dopamine, adrenaline, serotonin, GABA, acetycholine. The catechol and indole amines together constitute the major biogenic amines. These biogenic amines are found in great concentrations in certain parts of the brain associated with behaviour—namely the limbic system.

The levels of such chemicals found in the cerebrospinal fluid—the CSF-reflect the changes in brain chemistry. The experiments showed that, for example, the blood pressure reduced by an average of around 25%. The chemical levels in all those items measured changed to normal or near normal levels when tested after the yoga period was over. The levels stayed like this for at least 12 months after the yoga sessions were discontinued even amongst those who did not keep up the practise after the 6-9 month period

The epileptics experienced a substantial reduction in seizures, both in numbers and severity. The aggressive patients experienced a substantial reduction in aggressive episodes. All these groups had chemical tests performed regularly to discover the RATE of change and this seemed to coincide with the rate of reduction of the symptoms.

For some patients, there was no need to continue with drug therapy and for others for whom drug therapy was the next option they were excluded from the need for medication as a result of the success of the yoga study.

These studies are typical of those performed at various institutes in the West as well as India. The Himalayan Institute in USA has also been responsible for a vast array of experiments and controlled trials and the results have always been positive and have demonstrated continually that yoga therapy has a much more beneficial effect than any drugs—naturally without any unpleasant side effects.

The Himalayan Institute regularly prints the conclusions to these and sums up the results. Their basic statement is that local increases in blood supply to organs and glands produces more efficient working of the component. I would add that gravitional effects are also highly significant.

Lots of experiments on brain waves have also been conducted. In essence these show that the brain waves of the stressed person soon can be converted to the waves of the quiet mind by meditation. The alpha waves and beta waves increase whilst the theta rays decline which is interpreted as meaning stress has declined and the mind has become calm. There have been numerous experiments and all seem to point to the same phenomenon just described. One of these experiments was conducted upon a group of 25 people with a history of high blood pressure. The group was instructed only to perform shavasana, the corpse posture, in the following manner. Lie on the floor with feet spread 25inches and hands 10-12 inches away from the body. Focus on the sensitive parts of the body in turn and as soon as the mind is distracted move to another part of the body and focus solely upon this—and so on. This to be practised for 15 minutes a day for 6 months. The blood pressure was very substantially reduced, more so than the drug treatment of the other group. This was put down to reduction of stress. No other postures were used and no breathing practices—just the corpse. This trial was conducted by four medical researchers in Varanasi, India at the Institute of Medical Sciences at the Hypertension Clinic.

Datey, Patel and H.Benson conducted trials upon meditators with experience of TM—transcendental meditation as taught by the Maharishi Mahesh Yogi—and those people with normal blood pressure did not have any change to their blood pressure. Those who were hypertensive had a significant drop in blood pressure from above the normal back to normal over a 3 month period.

Further experiments upon zazen practitioners-Zen masters and other zen priests—show that the production of alpha waves is routine and with similar frequencies amongst the whole group of meditators whether in Japan or China. These waves were measured in the 4 main parts of the brain and alpha waves were produced in all 4 parts which it seems is very rare. Usually the theta waves are considered to be the result of intense mental activity and alpha waves are those of serenity of mind. Meditators seem to be able to produce the alpha waves at will and that would seem to be the point of the meditation effort. It seems that it is from this position of quiet mind that the valuable work of personal examination and introspection can be done.

9. Lungs and Lung Capacity

These need no introduction. Their function is obvious. Yet they are subject to much misuse in our culture, largely because we seldom fill them. In this regard yoga has no equals—the breathing practices ensure that complete breaths will be taken during the average session. What is the value of this? Let us see what happens during expansion of the lung tissue. The alveoli, the many broccoli-like structures branching off the main large pipes, the bronchii, are sacs which create the environment for oxygen exchange to take place. If you were to lay out the whole of the lung tissue, apparently it would take up the area of a tennis court—or is it a football pitch? No matter—it is a massive area. If the whole area can be used then the exchange of fluids through the tissue will clearly be more efficient the more of the area is exposed. How does yoga achieve this?

The most significant element of this process is the retention of breath—something that does not take place in normal life. Consider what the "kumbaka" phase of the breathing practices involves. You breath in for a specific count—say 6 seconds. Then the breath is held for, with some practice, 24 seconds which is followed by expulsion of air. The stale air that cannot be expelled –this is referred to as the residual volume of the lungs and is about half a litre for the average human being—will be diluted by this full in-breath. When this is expelled it is followed by a further dilution with the next retained breath. This continues until there is little trace of stale air. No amount of deep breathing in the Western way, will produce this effect because during exercise there is insufficient time for dilution to take place. This is unique to yoga.

Some of this stale air attaches to the major pipes –the bronchii—for the same reason as water flowing in a river moves very slowly by the banks but is at its maximum speed in the centre of the stream of water. By retaining the breath this slow moving air is also diluted and permitted to mix properly with the main body of air-thus the bronchii become subjected to full " cleaning" from the moving air, the eddies set up by the turbulent in-breath. This was fully understood a long time ago by the yogis.

We can consider all the other breathing practices involved in yoga but there are significant benefits that cannot be thought of as primarily value to lung function. We might consider kapalabhati as one of these practices. This involves fast abdominal muscle contraction, just as if one were intending to expel from the nasal passages, something like a fly. Whilst there is rapid air movement which must cause there to be a considerable increase in the movement of residual air in the bronchials, ---but not in the main body of the alveoli—it could be that the primary benefit physically is firstly control of function, which itself means that the person demonstrates mastery of a process—the main benefit may be vibration. The liver is strongly stimulated since it is directly attached to the diaphragm. In this regard, so must the stomach be. So the strong force of contraction produces waves of vibration across the whole abdominal contents. This low level vibration works like a pneumatic hammer when used to break up concrete—the constant application of force followed by withdrawal, causes strong vibrational waves which have a loosening effect upon all structures in the vicinity.

Dr M.V.Bhole states that the healthy person breathes more through one nostril than another and that this dominant nostril alternates every hour. Others have stated that it occurs about every 3 hours. The pressure changes or the increased velocity of the air-stream during alternate nostril breathing are seen to cause temperature humidity and other physical changes around the nasal mucosa which may stimulate nasal receptors and cause changes in pulmonary blood-flow with cardiac effects as well as changes in the size of lung airways.

High levels of CO_2 which develop during pranayama may cause an increase in the tolerance for CO_2 which will slow respiration and permit the person to be more tolerant of poor oxygen levels. What has also been shown by this researcher as well as others, is that increases in the oxygen levels in the blood which were expected to be revealed by the research were not so revealed. Swami Kuvalayananda, another prominent researcher in the science of yoga, surmised that the benefits must be seen as mental coming from the slow control of breath and not from oxygenation.

Asthmatics, according to Dr Bhole and others, are likely to benefit from pranayama because of strengthening of intercostal muscles which enables the sufferer to overcome the resistance created by the disease Bhastrika with forced quick expiration and slower inspiration creates a sort of venturi effect which is said to suck mucous from deep in the lungs and create expectoration. This same phenomenon is claimed to aid the draining of sinuses as well.

Hyperventilation from rapid deep respirations causes lowering of blood CO_2 levels and this leads to cerebral vasoconstriction and to slower unloading of oxygen from the oxygen carriers in the system— oxyhaemoglobin. The result is a relative deprivation of oxygen in the brain which is claimed to create spiritual effects. It seems that the researchers have also studied religions in other parts of the world, not connected with yoga, and found these pranayama practices inherent for the same reasons of spiritual stimulation.

It should be remembered that breathing practices have been designed to encourage prana not gaseous exchange. It is a regular part of my delivery to students that the real message of yoga is not physical but of course, this seed falls on stony ground until the aspirant already understands this herself. Until then most will primarily value the physical health benefits.

There will now follow a short synthesis of published research findings mostly from Indian medical and University research institutions.
Breathing Rate
One study on young fit people showed that there was a significant reduction in the number of breaths per minute from an average of 16.6 to 13.4 over the 6 months period of the study. The group was non-yogis who were taught the yogic practices.

10. Breath Holding Time

One researcher found that a group of newly taught yogis controlled against a group learning Canadian 5BX exercise programme and another group who did nothing special, increased their breath holding capability from 74.8 seconds to 99.3 seconds after 3 months of training.
Vital Capacity. The maximum average vital capacity is around 4.5 litres. Studies conducted by the prominent researcher Udupa, showed an increase of.91 in capacity as a result of a hatha yoga regime taught to a young group. This controlled study was carried out with a similar group of people doing the Canadian 5BX exercise programme and both groups compared with a control group. There was a.41 increase in the exercise group and no change in the control group who were given general walking and light exercise to do.
What was also noted was that vital capacity REDUCED after these groups were given fast running exercises to do. This may break an image for some people.

Looking at the pure anatomy of this region it is possible to observe from the surgeons dissection notes, that the heart creates slight indentations in the lung coverings so that it may be reasonable to assume that full expansion of the ribs has at least some direct mechanical effect upon the heart. Of course, if we look at kumbaka, the held in breath and consider the number of yoga pranayama practices that involve holding the breath and increasing the intrathoracic pressure by –usually--tightening the abdominal muscles while there is a full breath, it can be seen that the heart being in contact with the lungs and the lung internal pressure being increased dramatically by these practices inevitably affects the heart. Since there are numerous arteries and veins passing over the heart surface, beneath the outer fibrous layers attached to the diaphragm, it is again a reasonable assumption that this mechanical pressure from lung inspiration will squeeze these vessels and thus speed the flow of blood through them. This may have a beneficial effect on the prevention of arterial sclerosing or hardening of the arteries. This could be responsible for the reported reduction in heart troubles after taking up yoga—an improvement in blood flow via cardiac arteries.

11. Glands

Experiments at numerous institutes around the West and the East have produced a consistent result. That yoga practice benefits glandular function. The mechanism of this is considered to be great increases in blood flow. This occurs because of gravitational effects but also from compression during the postures. The alternating compression and decompression—indeed sometimes reduction in compressive force below the gravitational ambient such as can be achieved with uddiyana bandha, probably is responsible. Researchers speculate about this, as they do for the reasons for all the benefits of yoga, so my feeling is that my speculation perhaps is no less valid.

Studies in Indian medical establishments have consistently found a "normalising" effect upon glandular secretions. Of course, many of the studies have been conducted upon ILL people and many on those classified as not suffering from any identifiable medical condition. The implications of "normalisation" upon glandular secretion are interesting to speculate. Even though the subjects were classified as not identifying any medical condition, normalisation still occurred, strongly implying that many subjects were already mildly malfunctioning. Here we come, I believe, face to face with the absolute reality of yoga practice consequences---that yoga brings one back to what should be occurring within the body. This, if one is ready to accept it, suggests that the natural state for the human is stress free, well fed with proper food, with quiet contemplative time and time for rest and proper exercise. This could explain why children are generally healthier than adults. This also gives rise to my frequently made statement to thousands of yoga students –and indeed, to therapy patients, ---that yoga is designed to bring about a return of the child-like state. Dr A.M.,Moorthy who was assistant professor of physical education in a Madras college, conducted a trial amongst 180 boys and girls, equally divided by gender, in order to establish if, having learned and practised a yoga regime, a cessation of practise subsequently removed the benefits gained. He used a control group and conducted the experiment in accord with modern scientific demands. The results showed that after a period referred to as detraining during which no yoga was entered into, there was already showing reductions in the gains made. This is definitely in accord with my experiences. A fair number of patients have taken up yoga and found great benefits but when reappearing for treatment a year of so later, confess immediately to a cessation of the practices which led them to become pain free. It is usually lack of time that is put forward as the major obstacle, and it is probably almost invariably the person employed rather than self-employed. This is most likely to be pressure from colleagues. I have only one concrete example of this perhaps being incorrect and that is in a legal firm in which the partners instituted a yoga teacher to attend for the provision of yoga lessons once a week. One of these partners still complained about the difficulty of finding time even though the classes were held during company time, so it may be reasonable to assume that it comes right back to the individual. Not difficult to believe!

There are two readily identifiable nerve connections to the thyroid, for example. These are from C6 and C7, being adjacent to this gland. Thus it may be a reasonable assertion that interference with, especially, the latter, which is very common amongst patients, could interfere with thyroid function.

12. The Disease Process. How is it Cured by Yoga?

All the books from which I have included extracts agree –roughly speaking—upon the issues relating to the disease process at a local and cellular level. The osteopaths point to the micro trauma creating the inflammatory reaction which in turn creates a disturbance to the function of the joint involved. Nobody begins their analysis with the question— "why is there a micro-trauma"? Each in their own way states an example of how the micro-trauma could come about but each has left out a piece of understanding. Take the person who steps awkwardly off the pavement and " twists the spine". Why should this matter when the same person probably sat in his car seat the day before and twisted in his seat to reach round to take something off the rear car seat—and this without incident? Why should the pavement incident matter to a normal person ? My answer is plain. The disease/disorder/dysfunction syndrome is PRECEDED by a loss of mobility which is –generally speaking- symptomless. The writers all agree about the presence of an EVENT which creates the symptom. What is never recognised is what features are in place before the incident. It is the incident which is seen as the producer of the problem. There is no recognition of the real origin.

Consider teenage boys playing rugby. I have watched my own pulverise each other on the pitch and then walk off the pitch laughing and smiling and not—seemingly—injured. However, at 14 my youngest came away with a painful neck. I discovered that his trapezius muscle was very tight from forcing in the scrum—and years of computer games!!- and I treated this and there was no repetition. The mucles had become hard but were—relative to the severity of the problem—symptomless. The scrum in rugby had forced him to make a manoever that his tissue was not able to withstand.

I find the same characteristic in the vast majority of my patients. They state that a single event caused their problem—many times it is a completely innocuous event—but I can normally demonstrate that the charactistics for the successful failure of the tissue to be capable of withstanding the event were already well in place. We could look at men in a wrestling ring—how do they survive the assault? How do so many men survive the rugby field when it is plain that each takes a real battering during the game? The answer has to be that the body is ACCLIMATISED to the processes. It is able to accept the movements involved because the owner has acclimatised his own body to those demands. Thus if the rugby player were simply to run and twist to fend off another player as is common in the game and this twist caused an inflammation to a small part of his body he would be forced to stop and discontinue the game. This is a rare occurrence simply because the body is prepared. The person who steps off the pavement and jars his back is not prepared.

So—we look at acclimatisation. This really means that the stretching postures of yoga and the other normal activities of life—walking, cycling, swimming—is all that is necessary to prepare one for normal life. The fact that the body is flexible with yoga practice enables all the normal vascular processes to occur at each joint. It means that each joint has sufficient synovial fluid to keep it working correctly. It means that the muscles surrounding the joint are long enough to enable the normal movements of every day life to be accommodated without incident. It is the LOSS OF THIS ACCOMMODATION which gradually creates the loss of tissue integrity causing what is then referred to in the medical journals as pathology.

In the simplest of summaries—YOGA RESTORES NORMALITY. It does not produce abnormality.

13. Individual Yoga Postures – Analysis of their Effects

The preceding has been a series of statements about the overall effects of yoga. No researcher, as far as my own examination of a considerable quantity of published data has shown, has ever used only one posture and measured the effect of this, with the exception of corpse posture, shavasana.

All of the material I offer before entering into individual postural analysis has been designed to permit you to work out for yourself what is the benefit of each posture. In this regard, I make no claim that every benefit of all the postures is listed but I hope that you will " get the picture" and work more of it out for yourself. In this regard I am being my typical self and not spoon feeding my audience, but attempting to stimulate and encourage.

My aim now is to draw upon my own experience to weave a more intricate web for understanding the value. This web does contain genuine scientifically established facts, from experiments made by well respected medical researchers, but I have attempted to add strands from the following;

--the response from patients having no yoga experience who have been given one or two postures to perform as a way of assisting my manual work during the treatment phase
--patients attending the fmm clinic during training days who have been given posture to perform to assist in removing mechanical blockages

--" guinea pigs" regularly attending advanced remedial yoga workshops which I have conducted since around 1990, in several countries and over a wide range of samples of people

--students attending my own yoga classes who have requested assistance with immediately identifiable structural conditions ---for example Achilles tendon pain which often will decline quickly with a specific stretch which I have devised

--patients who have had acute attacks of minor musculoskeletal conditions and have telephoned me for advice, for which I have usually prescribed one posture to be done every day, just as if it were a pill!!

In this section let us take the popular postures and analyse what is happening. We will make what we hope will be helpful comments about the extent of each characteristic. For example, if we pick the forward bend as an example we will say that this will provide the maximum stretching of the posterior structures.

Headstand. Salamba Sirsasana

This is also known as rajasana, as well as its usual Sanskrit name, the inference being clear—it is the king of postures. Despite this, in the west today there is much prohibition of this posture and many fears about its performance. In our analysis we will simply state that which we know does occur and then make comment on these facts.

These details have been measured in yogis in experimental situations, in yoga hospitals and research institutions—they are not our speculation. During the headstand, there is a draining of blood from both legs and much of this ends up around the facial tissues, neck, arms and hands. This is entirely what one would expect. There is no increase in blood flow in the brain but –much more significantly—there is a redistribution. Those arteries which are being **well served** by blood flow send signals from the built-in baroreceptors—pressure receptors—to constrict the artery and reduce the quantity of blood. The **poorly served** arteries receive the opposite signal and open up to permit more blood. The results came from experiments using radioisotopes implanted and circulated around the arterial system.

This is the explanation given by the researchers for the increase in mental concentration and memory improvements. This characteristic has certainly happened to the author within months of taking up the daily headstand—even though it was poorly performed---and these improvements continue. In the case of the author there is no loss of memory due to age, something which in our culture is frequently spoken of as if it were an inevitability. As an aside, modern research—nothing to do with yoga –has demonstrated that brain function in a 90 year old is as good as in a 9 year old--- so as we suspected, brain quality does not fade because of increasing years—there is another much more sinister reason.—probably poor food which has become endemic to this country despite supermarkets and vast quantities of anything you want being available. In addition, if one has an open mind it is possible to observe that brain function loss such as occurs in Alzeimers Disease, is a peculiarly Western disorder and is virtually unknown in many societies, notably those in which old people are revered and who lead healthy lives.

As the veins in the legs close up whilst in the headstand, from blood pressure reduction and eventually full drainage of venous blood from both legs, there is a release of thrombin into the blood stream—surely this must be all the evidence we need that the creator intended us to perform headstands!! Thrombin is, of course, a natural anti-coagulant. The headstand is the only exercise known to humans in which the heart rate decreases whilst the calorie usage increases, which has led to the joke that the posture is a must for overweight people!! No one so far has come up with an explanation for this phenomenon.

The thyroid gland is engorged with blood and this increases the efficiency of the gland as well as flushing nutrient in greater quantities. This has been verified in controlled trials by Dhanaraj another prominent researcher in a major yoga institution-he demonstrated in a group as against an exercise group and a control group, that the yoga group newly trained, had significant increased levels of thyroxin in the blood within a couple of week of starting the yoga programme. The exercise group had a slight reduction.

The abdominal contents gradually drop down onto the diaphragm relieving pressure upon the femoral vascular structures. The adhesions surrounding abdominal organs will gradually be released as the headstand is repeated, until the organs move freely within the pelvic basin—this is the natural animal state and the most desirable state for humans since it means that there will be no interference to vascular and lymphatic supply to the fascial bags in which organs are suspended--- omentum is the common name for them. The animal on all fours, of course, has no organ compression since all organs hang from the spine, which itself is in the horizontal attitude. This is public enemy number one for humans— constant gravitational force on abdominal organs with its attendant disease propensity.

The draining of blood from legs provides the vascular structures with the opportunity to be infused thoroughly as soon as the position is reversed. This creates a rush of fluids within the pipes and tends to expand them just as a river swells after rain and clears dead wood from trees. This is a similar system of clearance—there is a daily purge, as one might call it. What worries most people about the headstand is not the position but the compression upon the neck---there is a pathological fear on the part of teachers that someone will harm themselves during the posture. So –first let us examine what actually happens at this part of the body.

Neck intervertebral discs do not have much opportunity to expand and compress as do the others along the spine because there is so little weight in the head. Lying down, therefore, has little decompression effect upon the neck. It is, thus, perhaps not so surprising that endemic to Western humans is spondylosis or spondylitis as it is more commonly called. In essence, this means that the vertebral discs are degraded by lack of movement—this is created principally by lack of nocturnal imbibition— this concept has been thoroughly explained in earlier parts of the book. If we can examine the headstand, therefore, not as a posture but as a powerful stimulant to a natural process that is inevitably interfered with by normal life, then perhaps it can receive better publicity.

There is another aspect of neck vertebrae that ought to be examined— this is the tortuous route taken by the vertebral arteries and veins—the numerous twists and turns of the pipework unavoidably create difficulties for the flow of blood—so anything we can do to make this passage easier should be welcomed. The headstand will create a considerable increase in the amount of blood that engorges the veins and arteries supplying the vertebrae. Whilst there is no blood supply to the intervertebral discs there is a normal supply to all the associated structures such as posterior and anterior longitudinal ligaments nerve trunks and fascia and small muscles.

The headstand is seen as a hazardous posture not, I think, because one is inverted, but more because of, firstly, the possibility of falling and hurting oneself and secondly the sheer force upon the head. This frightens many—for reasons which, frankly they do not themselves understand. Most, after reminding that they were always doing it during childhood without a thought, quickly point out that they were then young---and so on. What is plainly demonstrated is that the common perception is that age will make the person more fragile—perhaps this is the best word. The reality, of course, is that the human body is anything but fragile, at any age. The fascia alone has a tensile strength greater than mild steel. When people are told this they do not believe it is so tough-and that I suspect is because most have lost any contact with things that demand great toughness. The discomfort experienced upon performing the headstand is entirely normal and does not decline with time!! I have been practising almost daily for 20 years and it is as uncomfortable as it was when I began—the difference is that now I simply ignore the feeling. If the posture is performed by someone with a substantial thoracic kyphosis then there may well be repercussions so the student should first have good yoga experience before attempting the head stand. If the person is upright then the load on the discs is perfectly within the normal capacity of the disc to withstand the forces.

A regular question asked in yoga classes and workshops is simply put like this, generally speaking; "yes, but what about osteoporosis". Inherent in this is, of course, yet another thing to fear. There is no understanding that one might have osteoporosis simply because one has done too little—certainly it does not occur to those doing too much but appears amongst the weak and inactive.

Returning to the original theme of neck compression for therapeutic purposes, one is best to see the headstand as a complete health care system involving so many beneficial aspects that it is hardly any wonder that it is called the king of postures. This is the best basis for considering the posture-do not look at it as hazardous since if one is to consider hazards with which to compare it then begin with the motor car which kills 4000 people in UK each year, and causes severe injuries to 150,000. How many people do you know who have had an injury from the headstand—only the unconscious person, the unknowing, would avoid headstand because of a perceived hazard. The headstand is actually my barometer for the measurement of fear in people. On many occasions I have conducted a workshop and during the early part of the day have asked experienced teachers to perform the headstand and have listened to a barrage of excuses why it should not be done. It is a great test of mental strength and has a profound impact upon the individual's own self-belief. The fear of performing it is totally self-generated since it is physically very easy.

The spiritual benefits are harder to define since it is unlikely that it will be performed in isolation. However, there is a powerful feeling of contentment apparent during its performance and a feeling of satisfaction at the achievement. This has been said to me many times by those whom I pressed to attempt the posture. Each has remarked on what they perceive as the benefits. The teachers that I have taught, especially typify the best responses about this posture—many have visibly squirmed at my persistent chiding to at least try the posture and have then glowed all over –just lit up like a light bulb –when being able to show a competence in class, when previously there was fear. I am not sure that one can put a value on this other than to say "priceless". And that is how I sell it!!!

There is a further benefit, much harder to quantify. The head stand is a challenge to the fearful. It is a challenge to the ability to balance without falling. It is a challenge to the willingness to be discomforted.

In the head stand, especially when applying what is usually termed the beginners method with hands clasped(I have always used this method for my own practise favouring this above what is termed the advanced method) with practice one can either close the eyes or open them. Whichever is used it will be observed that there is no difference in the ability to balance. This is not the case when standing on both feet—now I presume that this is the case because those who begin the head stand practice regularly are usually in their 30's or older and have thus not done the headstand for at least thirty years—whereas standing on both feet is a daily occurrence and the person ALWAYS does so with eyes open. Now it is my contention that if the headstand is done with eyes closed it will quickly be realised that balance is unaffected and is not improved by opening the eyes. "So what"-- do I hear you say??—I believe that this phenomenon helps with general balance overall. This itself may stimulate you to permit more time to be spent in yoga with the eyes closed thus aiding mind calming.

The Cobra Posture. Bhujangasana.
If one were forced to offer just one posture which contains most value— an absurd concept of course—it would be the cobra. This is because it

attacks the most serious problem of the human being—the eventual destination for the old person, which is to be
stooped. It has to be remembered that the old - age stoop is very much a Western characteristic and comes not just because of old age but because ones physical labour is no longer wanted and of course, because of too much sitting. Being useful tends to reduce the depressive posture ---if you are no longer needed then old age can take its ravages easily, along with memory loss and brain fade!

The cobra causes the spine to round in the opposite direction. Let us see what actually happens.

The anterior longitudinal ligament which is as tough as a leather belt and three times as thick as its posterior cousin is the most significant obstacle to back bending. This characteristic is one indicator towards my strongly held conviction that we were supposed to be on all-fours and that we have poorly adapted. For the horse, this ligament is what prevents the rider from causing spinal collapse and it still exists in humans despite having no value. The cobra causes this to lengthen. The ligament is richly endowed with blood vessels and nerves and is what maintains the integrity of the forward parts of the intervertebral disc. The discs are heavily bound to the ligament so any opening at the front of the spine will create a strong stretch at the disc annulus. The annulus is highly fibrous, being constructed just as a car tyre with layers of tough material in various directions –actually following the construction of a radial ply tyre. The stretching creates a stimulus to the compression/decompression cycle which ultimately assists in the maintenance of the health of the disc. The amount of stretch which can be made to occur at the front of the disc is much more substantial than could be achieved by any other means—including traction and upside down suspension.

Cobra is, thus, fascially lengthening both the ligament and the abdominal muscles whilst this is also able to unpick the contracture in the diaphragm and its attachment to the ribs. The cobra gives the practitioner of yoga the opportunity, not available in any other physical activity, to expand the rib cage and stretch the fascia longitudinally as well as laterally. In other words, in both directions of contracture. This, however, requires skill and experience and is usually not what happens until several years have passed.

Cobra will engage the posterior spinal muscles, principally erector spinae group, in strong contraction and will maximally shorten them. Again, there is no comparable experience possible. This maximal shortening for a brief period, brings a great increase in blood supply and this is especially helpful for those who sit a lot. The increase in blood supply also helps to infuse additional repair materials in the surrounding spinal tissues. The cobra creates very strong compression upon the rear section of the IVD (intervertebral disc) once again engaging the compression/decompression cycle and thus helping to maintain the health of the disc.

The strong movement backwards, at some point, brings the spinous processes into contact. Once they are in contact there is then a system of leverage set up to facilitate stronger opening of the discs and further lengthening of the anterior ligament. This has to be accompanied, naturally, by more lengthening of the abdominal muscles, which are known as rectus abdominus. The strong compression of bone on bone strengthens the bone itself and is a non-damaging loading of bone to reduce the likelihood of porous bone. The next component to benefit from the increase of blood supply, is the nerve trunks as they emerge from the foramen, the" holes" created between two vertebrae. This will also stimulate additional lymph flow and movement of the lymph fluids along the spinal lymph ducts.

The vertebrae are bone covered by periosteum. The periosteum is richly endowed with nerves and blood vessels and the strong but gradual compression will increase the fluid flow at the micro- level as well.

Lying face down with the trunk raised will cause strong compression upon the abdominal contents and increases in organ blood flow will result. This will improve the function of the bowels, aiding elimination.

The neck vertebrae are also brought into closer proximity which will restrict the blood flow to the posterior vascular structures—arteries and veins –serving the neck area. This will increase the compression upon the posterior articulations and disc mobility will improve and blood flow to what is a heavily restricted area will improve considerably.

The use of strong contraction of lower spinal muscles during the active phase of this posture will bring much more blood to the sacral and lumbar nerve plexuses and this is cited by experimenters as being responsible for improvements in neurological quality—better balance, more accurate motor control, easier limb function.

The strong extension of the neck will enable stretching of the anterior neck structures to take place-notably the sternomastoid muscles and the scalenes and the frontal fascial envelope as a whole will be lengthened, reducing the pull inherent in the frontal fascial shortening which tends to pull the person into the stoop. The ribs individually will then be able more readily to elevate during proper breathing. This all helps to bring the person more towards the truly upright position.. The closer the person comes towards the physiologically upright position, the less the load on posterior muscles to maintain the upright position.

Cobra requires the tricep muscles to increase in strength --these will be the greatest beneficiaries in terms of muscle strengthening but others such as spinal muscles and trapezius will be stimulated in preparation for lengthening and proper stretching.

Intercostal muscle will of course, be lengthened by cobra and all the breathing practices will become physically easier as a result of back bending. The opening of the ribs at the front will create more fascia length in both sets of intercostals and create strong compression on the rib articulations at the vertebral connection.. This will improve the blood flow to that part of the vertebral articulation which is synovial. Being synovial it is subject to all the same strains and sprains and loss of movement that would occur to any joint such as a knee or elbow. Rib joints at the vertebrae are clearly meant to move just as are knees!

Cobra creates a strong stimulus to the heart and its associated pericardium to stretch, as the diaphragm is forced downwards during the cobra posture whilst the upper sections of the heart are attached to the neck and the sternum and thus will between them prevent the heart from travelling unencumbered downwards with the diaphragm. This also relieves the cardiac arteries many of which travel underneath the heart. Constant compression upon the cardiac arteries which is a feature of the lives of most people in UK as a result of sitting at work will, I believe, gradually reduce the amount of blood able to reach the heart. If you examine the posture of many men today, there is considerable thoracic kyphosis-rounding of the shoulders—which must restrict the amount of space for the heart. If this is the constant daily position and this remains unrelieved---obviously it must be so unless one has some form of back bending---then there will be constant interference to blood flow to the cardiac arteries which supply the heart muscle. This could be interpreted as further evidence of how poorly we have adapted to the upright position—of course, the quadruped will not have to suffer heart disease at least not from this source.

The cobra will also lengthen the aorta and vena cava, the two primary pipes for blood transmission to and from the lower body which will both be stretched in this posture. The aorta is subject -- in many men especially--- to bulges, which eventually burst—this is called an aneurism. Perhaps this results from too much interference to blood flow caused as indicated above. This is of course my speculation. But—what modern medics demonstrate beyond doubt is that they collectively have no interest in INVESTIGATING the reason for such things. There must be a reason— and this seems as feasible as any!

Cobra will enable some reasonable amount of stretching to take place along the rectus femoris –the fourth head of the quadriceps-- as it crosses the pelvis—this part is referred to as the superior anterior iliac spine—the ASIS—and it is almost unavoidable that there be some lengthening of the psoas, as well during the posture. It would be very hard to discriminate between the two elements during an observation of someone performing the postures, though.

Cobra allows the abdominal contents to hang from the spine—the natural vertebral state and may well be an aid to the process of removal of physical glueing -back again to adhesions!

In this posture the elevation of ribs and the consequent opening of lungs should enable deeper breaths to become a feature and with breathing practices, produce slower breathing with better regulation. Yogis long ago believed that the slower you breathed the longer you lived. This deduction was taken from observations of animals—elephants breath much more slowly than mice and live many times longer. We shall see!!

The arterial and venous blood flow in the neck vertebrae is capable of great restriction-this may add weight to my argument that we were intended to be on all fours because in this position the blood would naturally fall to this position—so that strong extension of the neck will produce stimulus to these structures whilst the frontal arteries, especially the carotid deep and shallow, will be stretched.

Intra-abdominal pressure will increase during the cobra increasing the blood flow within the abdomen. This increase will stimulate peristaltic action speeding up waste elimination, cited by yogic experimenters as the primary reason for bowel pathology.

You may have recently witnessed a Jamie Oliver programme in which he highlighted an average UK male and his quantity of faeces in comparison with the average Ugandan—the Ugandan was many times greater.

To summarise. There are so many benefits of practising the cobra –I have to say to you the reader that I have never before set them out in such detail and am amazed that there are so many and that they are so obvious when considering the construction of the human frame—that it behoves all yogis to ensure that this is never avoided. There is an increasing number of times that I see reference to avoiding, especially, neck extension and surely this brief dissertation on this one posture must persuade the most ardent critic within the yoga world at least to reconsider their view.

The cobra is cited as being responsible for black outs. It is technically possible for someone who has bony bits growing on their vertebrae for them to irritate a nerve or obstruct a blood supply pipe—but with so many benefits to avoid using this posture is equivalent to not driving your car on the grounds that you might have an accident. I have never witnessed anyone having this sort of difficulty with yoga nor during treatment. I have treated over 6000 people and taught yoga to at least 3000. I am considered to be a very strong and adventurous practitioner of physical therapy as well as yoga.—so do think clearly about the real risk. No cobra posture is going to threaten your health –no yoga posture can do this. The worst that I have witnessed or heard of is the person performing strong neck extension and feeling light headed after wards. The probable explanation for this would be some minor blockage to one of the vertebral arteries serving the brain or some part of the brain. But have faith that this vastly intelligent body could not be offended by anything invented by people of great intelligence so long ago and who have proved the system so thoroughly.

The forced extension of the spine during the posture, will compress the posterior surfaces of the sacro-iliac joints and will tend to normalise their function because during cobra and forward bend there is equal mobilisation in both normal directions of movement—although movement is so slight that it is not discernible to the uninitiated. This is especially important as a balance movement to strong forward bending. McKenzie in his book The Lumbar Spine states that in various USA studies of spinal function the loss of extension capacity is the most obvious and serious characteristic of normal people doing sedentary work. Cobra is the finest answer to this.

Because the sacrum tends to become strapped down so tightly with muscles shortening cobra is critical to the unpicking of this fascial strapping.

Forward Bend. –Paschimottanasana.
This is an equally valuable and powerful posture which also has a vast range of benefits-this should not be missed except in exceptional circumstances— disc rupture is the only occasion to be wary in this posture—in this case it should be performed standing in stead of sitting.
The most significant and valuable component is the lengthening of the fascial planes encasing the posterior muscles of the spine and the hamstrings. For the person with a stiff spine and short hamstrings this is absolutely vital as a posture and will dramatically transform the ability of the person to move with ease, sleep comfortably, get in and out of cars easily, play sport, walk and run—the list could almost be said to be endless!

The most frequent component of back pain, is contractured lumbar fascia and hamstrings. The combination of these two characteristics wrecks more bodies than any other single thing that is not classified as trauma. This is a slow death for the body and is the major component of "old age syndrome" with its consequences in the hip joints and knees.

The lumbar fascia is the thickest in the body and plays a critical role in supporting the muscles of the spine in their need to absorb shock, bolster the contraction capability, and provide a sort of supportive corset. This vital role also points to the downfall for many people because if this is not kept stretched and lengthened then the consequences of fascial shrinkage are greater than at any other part of the body. This is simply because of the sheer thickness of the muscle/fascia complex. The benefits of having such a construction are, then, great but are totally dependent upon proper maintenance. This is seldom achieved since so few understand what has to be done. Most consider that exercise is the answer—it is not; this is demonstrated by the quantity of professional athletes that come for treatment.

Holding the forward bend while the fascia stretches produces an immediate and tangible improvement in blood flow to the lumbar area. With shortened lumbar muscles comes a whole collection of by-products. The underlying muscle, the quadratus lumborum, is that which pulls down the 12th rib to enable full in -breath to take place. This muscle is attached to the pelvis, spine and 12th rib—when it is contractured it is impossible to be sure if this is what is wrong or whether it is the lumbar erector spinae and fascia that are at fault –but it is possible to deduce it if there is only one side in heavy contracture. Without forward bending quadratus lumborum would never fully lengthen. Because of its fascial connections around the rim of the posterior part of the pelvis, there is a reasonable chance that psoas would be affected. With this possibility comes a further possibility—contracture of latisimuss dorsi. If we construct this as a possibility then we have to add intercostals shortening as a further possibility. All these characteristics are affected in the forward bend though my extensive experience with low back treatment with subsequent yoga leads me to say that yoga would take a long time to create the full elasticity of tissue at this part of the body in some people, these being big men with massive stiffness. Ex –rugby players would be the first to qualify!

However, to make an accurate diagnosis is beyond all but the most experienced physical therapist although the experience advanced yoga teacher such as the ones I have taught would be competent to see this characteristic.

We are holding the forward bend. The possibility is that the most unpleasant part is the pain at the back of the knees—this is short hamstrings!. The hamstring fascia and gluteal fascia are interwoven and thus end up weaving with the lumbar fascia—hence the value of the forward bend because it will stretch the complete envelope from head to toe-literally. Because the hamstring fascia which envelopes each muscle belly runs from the pelvis to the knee, this posture has a greater effect than any other.

The latissimus dorsi muscle—I use the shortened term lats--- is also heavily stretched by this posture and it too is an important component of back pain. The short lats draw down the arm and prevent the torso from having full movement—the forward bend will begin the process of stretching of the lats but there will need to be supplementary postures to make the process complete. Remember that latissimus dorsi is attached to the upper arm and to the pelvis—so literally your arm is attached to your pelvis. In the forward bend another serious problem is tackled thoroughly. The stiff spine and short hamstrings create nerve trunk compression and adhesions at certain parts where guider straps are placed. All the major joints have places where the nerve trunks are held in place-these are called retinaculae—this is like a cable clip in an electrical system, except that the cable clip prevents the cable from moving whereas the retinacula simply provides the mechanism to prevent the nerve cable from being displaced to the inappropriate position—so nerve trunks should be able to move freely by sliding underneath the retinacula. If there is no lengthening for many years, the retinacula becomes the cable clip preventing movement and this then becomes a site of some symptom. It is my theory that this is the real explanation for Carpal Tunnel Syndrome.

This can mimic the symptoms of a disc rupture, a disc bulge, muscle contracture, trigger points---much misdiagnosed by all manner of physical therapist.

The nerve trunks will be strongly tractioned through the spinal foramen as they emerge from the spine and pass down the legs- if the toes are drawn towards the head whilst performing the posture, this creates the maximum possible lengthening of the nerve trunks. The lymph channels and ducts will be similarly stimulated.

The ribs will swing towards the closed position and there will be maximum stretch at the posterior intercostal muscles. The spinal cord will receive a strong stretch as well, provided the head is kept down and with force applied at each end of the cord there will be an unpicking of any adhesions along the way. Spinal cord adherence at three points in the full length is sometimes cited by physicians as reasons for pain.

Blood vessels, particularly the femoral arteries and veins, will get direct stretching force tending to straighten any kinks in the pipes. This itself will encourage better flow. Since the blood vessels travel down the fascial clefts -this probably accounts for much of the general discomfort which hamstring shortening brings—there will be less adhesions and thus more freedom of movement of both nerve trunks and vascular structures. There is around a 2cm excursion of nerve roots between the vertebrae during the forward bend when performed to the maximum range-head to knees.

When the posture has improved to the point at which the chest approximates to the knees—this usually takes a few years—the compression upon the abdominal organs will be considerable. There will be strong force applied to the adhesions between organs as well as more blood forced into the organs. The mechanical compression effects of the posture will improve the bowel function both stimulating peristaltic action and mechanically extruding waste products. Naturally this is controllable!!

Hip muscles such as piriformis are affected by the posture though there are more powerful postures which have a greater effect. There is some effect upon the calf muscles but again this is not as much as given by other postures. The maximum stretching effect is, thus, upon the posterior structures and nerve trunks.

For the person who has had a reliable diagnosis of IVD rupture or bulge—only an MRI scan can do this reliably—this posture should be replaced by the forward bend performed standing. In this position the disc is not under compression and as soon as the person is able to perform the posture with the spine brought below the horizontal position—this is as soon as the hamstrings are long enough to permit this—then the disc is placed under traction and thus tends to draw in any bulge in the disc. This element makes it critical in any case of sciatic pain in which the sufferer feels symptoms in either foot, to comply with this statement and avoid the seated forward bend. Otherwise it should be performed by all and strongly---but especially this posture—with sensible caution and gradually. I have seen several cases of young strong men— rowers who had come for treatment—straining the sacral ligaments because they failed to take due note of my strictures not to work too hard at the forward bend for several years at least!!

Nerve root adherence has been mentioned several times. Adherence also occurs to the nerve trunks which are the cables that pass down through the body. They will adhere at the retinaculae and by direct compression as they pass through the fascial clefts and are thus subject to the effects of muscle broadening which itself results from contracture.

Classically this posture is seen as being complete when the trunk rests on the thighs and the toes are pulled towards the head by both hands. This latter part of the posture produces lots of pain for many students and should really be included with the greatest circumspection making wise use of gradual introduction of this part. This should not be seen as a failure to perform the posture if this part has to be avoided because nerve trunk pain on stretching is too great.

It has always been a source of curiosity to me that powerful forward bending does not remove erector spinae contracture. The hard indurated tissues of the paraspinal muscles do not get soft and deltoid-like, performing the forward bend. I do not know why this is. If a very heavily built man has had many years of rugby in his youth and comes to yoga with tight hard indurated erector spinae, and of course is complaining of pain, then the pain will almost certainly be gone within one or two months. Now this would raise the question—which structure caused the pain—plainly it is not possible to be sure of this as even deep work into the muscles during fmm will not guarantee that no other structures are affected. Indeed, one expects to influence other structures even though the attempt is made to isolate the source of pain as being in erector spinae and thus working on these muscles removes the pain thus inducing in the mind of the patient that there can be no other possibility.

Looking at many MRI scans of the lumbar spine, it is plain that there are few patients with absolutely no problems what so ever. It is general for there to be something to report upon and this always means that there is SOME pathological change. If we are agreed that the PRIME reason for this is congestion produced by too little movement then we must make the spine move to a point not previously possible. Let us look at what structures are preventing full movement at this part of the body. The finest diagrams showing this appear in The Physiology of the Joints, Kapandji.

There are substantial ligaments holding L5 especially, to the pelvis and the sacrum. The diagrams of this part of the body show clearly the huge size of the tendonous part of the erector spinae as it passes across the L5/sacrum area, underlying which are the ligaments referred to. This is the greatest " bundle" of fascial tissue anywhere in the body and even if for no other reason, this is the reason for not avoiding the forward bend. Without this posture, this area of the body will progressively congest, the fascia will thicken and toughen, compression from the forces of contracture will increase and thus interference with the water imbibing mechanism will take place. There is no other rational interpretation of the reasons for the massive number of Westerners suffering with degeneration at this spinal level and it fits perfectly with the evidence from my own therapy practice.

Interestingly, there is a current patient who typifies this. He is 50, is very fit and active and has no medical history. He has suffered with back pain, what the medics would call ""non-specific back pain" for over a year and has had every means of physical therapy tried on him. As a last resort he went to see a spine surgeon who pronounced, from observing his MRI scan, that there was nothing wrong other than a bit of " normal wear and tear|" (please do read my remarks about this ridiculous phrase). The surgeon, thus, said he could not help. On examination, I found several joints seized up but freeing them did little to ease the pain. What produced an immediate loss of pain and the feeling of complete freedom was to discover the erector spinae muscles at the base of the spine to be rock hard, and to work deeply into these. One treatment session produced 50% improvement. The surgeon called what he saw on the MRI " normal wear and tear". Regrettably this does nothing to enlighten the patient—what it does do is reinforce the idea of age being the dominant factor. Looking at the rest of the spine and seeing that it is not affected as are the two bottom vertebrae should engage the diagnostician in thinking that age cannot discriminate within the same body—surely? But as the famous Dr. Cyriax has repeatedly said of his own kind, logic is not part of orthopaedic medicine.

How does pain come from the contractured myofascial network? This is simple—it is another case of congestion and failure to eliminate metabolic wastes adequately.

We return to the issue of the forward bend. This posture is widely condemned, even within the Pilates system. We could make the same remark as the famous doctor—that logic is also not part of physical therapy or exercise|.| If it were then everyone would undertake yoga, indicating that they DO understand how logical it is. Pigs will fly when this happens.

I have engaged—foolishly it turns out—in discussions on this issue with Pilates teachers but none have been willing to deepen the debate and prefer to carry on as they are without further examination. That is their right because to see the logic would force them to recognise the absurdity of so much of what is classed as systemised exercise.

The powerful forward bend has another strong benefit, not available from any other activity. Sacro-iliac joints are the connection between the sacrum and the pelvis, this being classed as a rudimentary joint until relatively recently. It is now considered to have synovial activity. About 100 years ago medics stated that it did not move and therefore could not be a source of pain because it could not dislocate. It is now recognised – although not in medical circles generally—that it could be the source of considerable pain and can mimic the pain of sciatica. I have seen enough in my own therapy practice to need no convincing(although the incidence is probably one in 500). If the forward bend is performed then all those fascial and ligamentous bindings around the sacrum and ilium will be given the elastic stimulus which comes from holding a posture. This will enable the sacrum to tilt in its normal mode something which will progressively be lost in age unless it is retained in this way. The immobility of the sacrum comes with the territory of increasing immobility which again is identified with the ageing process. I

have found loss of sacral mobility and loss of lumbar lordosis to be much more common than the one in 500 –this all can be corrected with yoga postures,; of course, not just with the use of one posture since equally strong back bending is needed.

There is one other aspect of forward bending which deservers an airing. The fascial bag running over the feet, calves, hamstrings, gluteals and eventually the back, has a powerful tractive effect upon the pelvis when it is contractured. Short hamstrings are endemic to the culture and can be witnessed in infant schools. The fascia weaving through the hamstrings and gluteals has a strong tendency to pull the pelvis backwards, creating the stimulus for the lumbar spine to lose its lordosis with consequent increase in the thoracic kyphosis. The result of this is the stoop of age. This tractive force cannot be felt nor witnessed only deduced, The clue comes from poor performance of the cobra and cobra should be used by guides and teachers as a major diagnostic tool to see this characteristic occurring. If the pelvis tilts it will create the need for the erector spinae to keep active to prevent the loss of lumbar lordosis—thus the erector spinae will compensate for the increasing tractive effect of shortening hamstrings. It does not require much brain power to see that this situation has to be broken if the person is not to become effectively old.

Side Bending. Parighasana.- variations of this.

This is performed kneeling with one knee on the floor and the other leg outstretched to the side. The arm on the side of the bent leg should then be taken overhead and used to aid the force of side bending. Immediately one attempts the posture for the first time, the place where the pain is felt is at the open side as the arm goes overhead. The latissimus dorsi is, in this posture, given the maximum opportunity to lengthen and the posture produces the strongest possible lengthening force of any posture. The most affected structures are lats followed by corset muscles—at least, two of the three muscles constituting the corset will be strongly affected. These are external and internal oblique muscles which form two of the three parts of the corset—the third is formed by the transversalis muscle which is formed rather like a cummerbund as worn during evening dress. To some extent this will also be stretched but since the fibres run around the waist the maximum effect upon transversalis is reserved for other postures.

In this posture there will be very strong compression upon the " closed" side which will heavily influence blood flow in the major organs juxtaposed—the liver in the case of a right side bend and the stomach in the opposite direction. The intercostal muscles will also be very strongly stretched and in this posture it will be possible to ensure that the fascial layers over the ribs are given maximum traction, once again giving the overall "plastic bag" a good chance to end up loose and free.

Adductor muscles receive a strong stretch in this position –for some people—but this very much depends upon the general flexibility of the person. For those new to yoga this should be a very significant addition to the postures for this reason alone. The hip joint seldom receives a demand to move to this position so there is a valuable effect upon the ligaments of the joint as well as the capsule surrounding the joint. Hip joint immobility is endemic to our culture now, probably as a result of so much sitting in cars and behind desks, and one major contributor to this situation is shortening of the adductors on the inside of the thigh. The posture provides a relatively easy way of beginning to lengthen them. Knee pains are frequently caused by short adductors and hamstrings. Once again the nerve trunks will receive strong traction and blood flow to all the femoral structures will improve, generally affecting circulation to feet as well.

The thoracic inclination will provide strong mobilisation to rib articulations with the vertebrae, one of the few opportunities for such force to be applied to this usually immobilised area. Again nerve trunks will be pulled strongly on one side. The neck vertebrae will receive strong side bending as well.

Adhesions of organs to ribs and the underside of the diaphragm will strongly be pulled away in this posture on the open side and of course very powerfully compressed upon the other side. The key to health of organs is that they are kept mobile and free of adhesions.

The side bends performed as described will principally affect the external and internal oblique muscles –which with the overlying transversalis I named the corset. The corset when it has shortened, is responsible for a great many back pain episodes and has been found, when stretched in rotation, to yield almost magical cure results. The corset is a major component of pelvic freedom something not much in evidence in Europeans. This may explain why Eastern people have always danced and these dances often require pelvic mobilisation—belly dancing, flamenco and so on. In order to perform these dances the pelvis must be free to move in relation to the spine—the corset if it is soft and long will enable this to occur.

A favourite place of strong adherence is at the scapula. The attachment of latissimus dorsi at the upper arm necessarily creates heavy congestion around the scapula, something which fmm therapists constantly discover. The teres muscles, the serratus posterior, lats and infraspinatus all become fascially bound up and this is one of the factors contributing to the postural stoop on the dominant side. Many right handed people display a right shoulder which is lower than left and this can usually be seen to be caused by the above characteristics. The side bends performed strongly will gradually remove the heavy contracture of the relevant muscles bringing with it much more freedom of scapula movement which will itself ease the load upon the horizontal fibres of the trapezius, especially, since it is these fibres that do the work of holding up the shoulder against the resistance created by downward-pulling latisimus dorsi. The lats will, because of their generous fascial covering, also restrict the ribs over which they move—again we come across adhesions.

Observing someone perform the side bend—this is really a gate posture performed in a particular way and not really the way shown in yoga books—it is relatively easy to see if either hip is troubling them. Short adductors will be very obvious since generally the knee will be forced to bend as a consequence of shortened adductors.

This is another of those posture not to be avoided whatever the reason. If it cannot be done kneeling on the ground then it should be standing. For maximum effect whether kneeling or standing, ensure that the hips do not rotate and are kept properly in line with the outstretched leg.

The force required to ensure gradual fascial elongation along the whole lats range, is substantial and will be most unpleasant.

Seated Spinal Twists. Ardha Matsyendrasana.

This choice of posture to form part of every day practice is essential because it influences everything. If you consider the juxtaposition of two vertebrae with the interposed disc, it can be seen that putting this structure into a twist will tend to shorten and compress each disc. This phenomenon can be mimicked in wringing a towel. Gradually with increasing turning there will be shortening of the towel and powerful force of stretching of the tissues on the outside of the structure whilst heavily compressing the inside section. There will be a heavy force applied and the discs will be compressed strongly giving stimulus to the natural compression/decompression cycle. It is this posture which I believe gives most value to yoga –and that may be because it affects everything.

The abdominal organ compression and twisting adds further power to remove adhesions and improve blood flow. The neck is a frequent component of general stiffness—this posture if it combines neck rotation as it should, can transform a person from a stiff old person to one able to perform normal tasks without pain, within one year.

Because it is performed first one direction and then the other, it tends to have a more powerful effect upon structures. For example, the trapezius muscle around the shoulders is almost invariably contractured and the twist will cause one half of it at a time to be strongly stretched. But only some of the fibres will be affected so that to fully stretch trapezius, requires the plough posture as well. Even this does not substantially affect the horizontal fibres of this muscle

In McKenzie's The Lumbar Spine there is some discussion as to the origin of much back pain being the result of over stretching on rotation and thus causing strain or what could be classed as genuine tissue injury. This "injury" is then mildly "demonised" whereas, once again, the medical mind has not grasped the real reason. Once a person is stiff and rotation is seriously restricted, which in my therapy practice is very seldom not the case, trying to rotate to achieve some physical task that the body perceives as not possible, will result in tissue tearing. This will repair but will result in the congestive/ inflammatory condition I have described. So the real reason is loss of mobility, not the action which was seen to precipitate the injury. I do not use the word injury unless I see clear evidence of trauma because what I have described above is not a primary but a secondary—in other words, the injury is the result of some other much more powerful force—gradual and imperceptible loss of myofascial range. There, of course, lies the explanation for so few people being able to see it. It is imperceptible to anyone other than the rare few who can see what is happening to them.

The seated spinal twist will progressively restore the range of movement, lost as a result of myofascial contracture. This has been demonstrated in my therapy practice, my yoga classes and the practices and classes of all those I have taught so there is a great wealth of evidence of the accuracy of this statement.

Seated spinal twist affects every part of the spine. No part is left unmoved but it should be recognised that this posture does not maximally affect any one part. What it does do is to ensure that nothing is excluded from its effect and in this regard it is unlike all postures.

We can see that the upper spine will be greatly affected but that the lower lumbar will not be as significantly affected. This posture is useless as a preventive for L5 seizure since it will not reach this lowest level. To reach the lowest lumbar level in twisting requires a lying down spinal twist, performed in a manner requiring to be modified from a yoga posture. The nearest equivalent is seen as a general twist moving both legs over from one side to another. It can simply be shown that this does not have any effect on the vast majority of people, down at the lower part of the spine. It is a reasonable general twist but lacks the power of the seated twist, because in the seated version it is possible to apply great force through the use of both arms in leverage. This lying down twist, to be effective at L5, must be modified by taking the lower leg right back as far as it is possible to place it, and then performing the twist. This really requires personal supervision from someone who knows how to do it.

Not just spinal articulations are heavily compressed by this move but corset muscles are lengthened. This is the other great value of the lying down twist. This group of three muscles has a lot to answer for. It is not enough to mobilise the spinal vertebrae without recognising the huge importance of this group of muscles. There are other posture to achieve this as well.

The nerve trunks are living structures just as are all other human tissues and need to be treated to mobilisation. They are sent to emerge via the foramen formed between the two arches of two juxtaposed vertebrae. Even though the space through which the nerve trunk emerges is many times greater than the thickness of the nerve trunk itself, the frequency of nerve root compression is substantial. This comes as a result of discs bulging and bits of disc breaking off and jamming against the nerve root as well as herniation of discs. Also. Surgeons report cleaning out these spaces during surgery to remove what I describe as "gunge"—probably detritus and congealed lymph. What is demanded of all structures is that they are moved so that the spinal twists will tend to traction the nerve roots thus having a sort of drain- rodding out effect. The strong traction on the nerve root should pull it further through the foramen and at certain points in the spine this excursion is around 2 cm. This is not a microscopic amount but measurable with a ruler!! This measurement has been made using Lasegue's test otherwise known as the straight let raising test. This test is often applied by surgeons and other orthopaedic specialists when conducting a spinal examination. It does not embrace the full lengthening of the spinal nerve roots so that the actual excursion of the nerve root could be twice that length—but this is entirely my speculation.

In the seated spinal twist, if it is done with both knees bent rather than one leg held straight, the power that can be generated by the leverage mechanism—the arm around the knee and the hand on the floor—will provide an opportunity to strengthen muscle. But this strength of twisting that is possible in this position will bring the rib cage to be rotated more than any other position could achieve. Again, this brings a likelihood of further deep breathing improvements and in this position it is possible to learn well how to control the length of breath.

In the seated spinal twist, if performed with both legs bent, the hips are affected strongly. If the right leg is over the left, then the gluteal group on the right hip is likely to be powerfully affected and it may be possible for the practitioner in this position to affect the deep ligaments posteriorly. These will be femoral ligaments encasing the head of the femur. With the under leg, the hip will be abducted and the power of stretching will be in the direction of external rotation. Indeed, watching a patient or yoga student perform this posture one is presented with much diagnostic data about the state of the spine and hip joints, perhaps the two most heavily affected parts of the body in musculoskeletal trouble.

The primary reason for the stricture to hold the spine erect in this posture is to ensure that the effects of rotation are directed wholly at this mode rather than partially dissipated in forward /side bending. One can witness many practitioners being asked to keep the spine upright but they have usually not been told how or why.

Fascial binding of the diaphragm to the ribs and abdominal muscles is very common. This creates poor function of diaphragm. If you ask a 5 year old child to hold up his arms above his head the brings his hands together above his head you will be able to observe that the lower part of the ribs swings outwards making a conical shape of the torso. Ask the average adult to perform the same movement and you will be able to observe that the lower ribs barely move and that the conical shape is inverted!!. That is, the upper part of the ribs is wider than the lower part—this is not how it is supposed to be. The child state is how it is supposed to be—this child state indicates that the abdominal muscles and diaphragm are operating separately and do not adhere to one another. The adult state indicates that adherence is complete. This has occurred for the very simple reason that prevention has not been undertaken.!! Weight training may have much to answer for here.

The combination of spinal twist and back bends will eventually free this part of the body, enabling correct breathing to take place. By the act of liberation of the diaphragm from fascial binding, easier and more efficient breathing will ensue as a matter of course.

Camel Posture. Ustrasana

This is one of the finest yoga postures for discovering where you are on the physical path to recovery and full movement. This sorts out the wheat from the chaff, as it were. The benefits are substantial in number and I will enumerate them. Top of the list is the opening of the chest, reflecting an opening of the person. It is the position of great openness, great vulnerability. One needs faith and trust because of the unusual nature of the posture. If it is done with the hands resting on the feet and with the hands turned out rather than in, then the maximum stretching value across the upper part of the chest, including pectoralis major, will ensue. In this regard for most people it is a particularly demanding posture. With the head held back and the hands turned out there is a strong stretching of the fascia which coverrs the whole of the frontal neck and upper chest area. This area when it is shrunk—as it is with rounded postural " stoop"---continually drags down the head towards the feet, successfully maintaining the head forward and flat chest posture, the posture of depression. The camel is your exit strategy from the posture of depression!.

The posture also presents the finest opportunity to unpick the fascial knotting around the diaphragm. It is the most appropriate posture for this difficult task. The need for this to occur can be seen plainly when watching someone who is not adept at this posture. Study the width between the lower part of the ribs as the person is in the posture—in the child like state, there is a wide gap between. In the person who has poor posture or who has spent a lot of time bent over a desk there is almost certain to be a narrow gap. The cobra posture will, of course, be the early start to the unpicking of this immobile part of the body but the fascial stretching will only take place in one plane. This is head to toe—there will be no lengthening across the fascial plane from left to right. The use of the camel posture will enable the student to get at this part of the restriction by using a strong in-breath whilst holding the posture. With practise it will become possible to open the upper abdominal area using this posture. Do remember that this is an adepts posture and what is described will take a few years to master.

A further place of great restriction for many, is the attachment of the rectus femoris muscle over the frontal part of the pelvis. This is known as the anterior superior iliac spine—ASIS for short—and years of hard physical sport, especially cycling, tend to make this an area of heavy fascial binding. The camel will aid the removal of the fascial binding but it is not the posture with the most strength for achieving this. The prize for this has to go to reclining hero.

There are few other additional benefits of camel. Spiritually, it is best seen as a powerful opening out posture, assisting the awakening process because of the strength of the spinal extension. In this regard it is superior to the cobra but the cobra is best seen as the starting point and the camel seen as the next rung on the ladder towards openness.

For many years this is a hard posture and imposes strong discipline upon the practitioner of yoga—especially if it is performed against great physical resistance and with mental reluctance—which is common!
Indeed, it is the most powerful posture for this area, this stretch not occurring at all in the cobra posture since the arms are held by the side of the body and pectoralis is not affected.

The most value in this posture comes, in my view, from two things. Firstly, the neck extension brings the cardiac fascial attachment further away from the heart which moves away from the neck as a result of the diaphragmatic excursion towards the feet—that is to say that the heart is lengthened literally, enabling the pericardium to be stretched. This is my view that pericardium is subject no less to fascial shrinkage than any other structure. Expanding the fascial envelope again will give the heart more freedom and space at the very least enabling the cardiac arteries to be relieved of compression. The contrasting forward bend –maximum compression upon the heart—and camel which creates maximum lengthening of the heart-- will create huge forces of liberation to be applied to the heart and its associated structures. This will satisfy the basic laws of living that compression and decompression must occur regularly.

The camel which involves the head being taken back, has created a lot of controversy, largely because of this latter fact. I conducted an experiment once, during a workshop for 20 experienced yoga teachers. All the teachers were asked to perform the camel. Only a few approached it without hesitation, several refused and others were reluctant. One lady said that she did not do this posture because taking her head back had a bad effect. I asked her to lie on a nearby desk with her head right at the end of the desk. The group and myself gathered round. I asked some group members to slide her body along the desk until the head would fall off the end of the desk but assured her that I would support her head in my hands and would not do anything to her head. She accepted this and remained like this whilst I assured her that I was continuing to hold the head but that I was now going to very slowly lower the head but that she could stop anytime. The group members now began to nod in understanding. Gradually I let go until her head was hanging off the desk unsupported—the neck was thus in virtual full extension. She stated that all was fine and waited for me to explain what was going on—the group members had now realised that this lady was not only lying with her head hanging inverted but the neck was fully extended—much more so that in the camel.

Now I asked her to perform the camel and agreed to support her head whilst in the posture which she did. Again I held the head and then gradually let it go and she declared that all was well –there were no ill effects. She eventually admitted that her own teacher 20 years before had strongly advised avoiding the camel posture—this showed to me and the group the power of suggestion. She was now assured that all was well and declared that she would be performing this posture because of the many benefits!

The point of the story is that FEAR creates so many obstacles that are unreal-they are simply figments of imagination and yoga should remove them—but one has to be very aware of ones own fears first—and when teachers inhibit students they do them the most weighty disservice.

One argument put forward for not performing this posture, is knee pains and the difficulty in kneeling while the posture is performed. This in itself should not remain a bar—one can find some form of padding to place under the knees and at least a poor attempt can be made by first sitting upon the heels and then with hands on ankles an attempt made to come up into the posture even if it is only for a few seconds. This establishes as a minimum, the intention to make the posture part of your routine. This intention has great value.

Just as the cobra enables the practitioner to decongest the diaphragmatic fascia so does the camel but there are different layers and levels which are presented in this posture, largely as a result of the arms being turned out stretching the chest fascia. This is why the head back position is critical to the value of the posture since the head back position takes the superficial fascial planes and fully exposes them to lengthening right down to the pubic symphisis.

This posture enables the person to use the full in- breath during the posture to fully open the lower ribs out till they become as they are with the child—very wide. This does take extraordinary force and determination and will take many years to achieve.

Camel and cobra are the preparatory postures for the wheel posture and it would seem appropriate to consider this posture now

The Wheel Posture. Chakrasana
In this posture what can be experienced physically is a powerful stretching force down the length of the linea alba which runs from the base of the sternum to the pubic symphisis. This line of tendon can be felt to be one of the primary restrictors of back bending even though you may not have felt it in either of the two preparatory postures. This characteristic can now be felt because this is the only posture in which the whole frontal fascial envelope is stretched. Of course the rear structures are readily tackled in the forward bend but there is no other opposing equivalent. Camel approaches it as does cobra but neither engages the whole body-only wheel does this.

Most people in yoga do not aspire to be able to perform this posture but when you do manage it there is something tremendously celebratory about reaching this point—one might say it is the pinnacle of achievement. Of course, soon after you reach this stage this feeling gives way to the realisation that anything is possible. This is precisely what one wishes to achieve with yoga postures—the freedom from restriction and symbolically the wheel gives you this in great measure. I have been with many students and more advanced practitioners when they have said that they would never be able to perform this posture—and then did so within a short period!

The posture itself has little physical value beyond the obvious—it cannot do any more than the cobra and camel except the little extra stretching of frontal structures. It will produce more strength in the arm muscles and is most valuable as a diagnostic tool. It will help you to decide whether an inability to perform it is due to spinal stiffness or weakness in arm muscles thus enabling you to work on those aspects of your practice that will gradually produce an ability to perform the posture.

 If you do wish to verify the obstacle, first perform the plank as described below and then the camel and it should be easy to see which of these two aspects of your body is dominating the failure to come up into the wheel.

The Plank Posture.Dandasana

As its name implies this is a posture which involves lifting the straight body off the floor using, principally, the triceps. The body begins face down with the hands placed by your side in such a way that the forearm is perpendicular to the floor. This dictates that the upper arm is horizontal and in turn ensures that it is principally a triceps strengthener. There will be other shoulder muscle strengthening takes place as well. The primary benefit is to the triceps but it presents an opportunity to demonstrate determination to hold a posture even in the face of an obvious inability to perform it fully. The mind concentration and focus on the breathing during the posture make it a great posture for mental strength.

Holding the arm muscles in maximum power will occlude the arterial and venous blood flow for the period of performance of the posture and the release from the posture will create a considerable effusion of interrupted blood flow into the poorly served tissues, rather like cleaning out all the ditches in the farmers fields allowing unrestricted fluid flow. This characteristic is not peculiar to the plank posture and does occur in all postures in which maximum muscle contraction is held for the duration of the posture. The effects are the same anywhere in the body. The build up of blood pressure in muscles produces the facility to flush the pipework through preventing stagnant blood and lymph which is cited in ancient medical systems as one of the major contributors to disease. Yogis understood that infusing tissues with a steady supply of blood would ensure good health and that restricted flow would lead to the breakdown of the normal repair and maintenance processes which the body is so well able to create—given the absence of restrictions in the form of muscle contracture especially. You will have read earlier on that this view is held by modern osteopaths as well.

The build up of blood pressure during the holding of any strong posture, which is concentrated within the muscles doing the hard work, creates a sort of damming effect with a strong restriction in flow. The build up of pressure in the muscles undergoing maximum contracton will be released immediately the posture is stopped. This phenomenon can be felt as a hot feeling within the area and improves the efficiency of vascular flow by opening up the pipes which may be poorly functioning.

Plank should be seen substantially as a means of strengthening the will since many an ancient sage has said that this is the weakest muscle in the human body. I tend to agree with this.

The Warrior Posture. Virabhadrasana

Warriors are primarily here for strengthening. They do this by demanding the practitioner hold the posture as strongly as possible. If we take the traditional warrior with the arms held above the head and hands together, then the posture presents some very valuable characteristics. Firstly, the forward thigh muscle should be held horizontal which itself will present the opportunity to gradually strengthen the thigh muscle. Secondly it obliges the practitioner to consider how to raise the arms directly overhead with hands touching but not clasping whilst placing the trunk facing forward and preventing rotation. This is

one of the greatest postures for teaching the practitioner the art of what I call "differential relaxation". The act of holding the arms overhead requires the ability to allow the scapulae to rotate since half of this movement is permissible because of scapulae rotation but the trapezius is the muscle principally involved in the creation of this movement. The latisimuss dorsi is attached to the upper arm and runs down to the pelvis. Some parts of this muscle are needed to cause the trunk to come upright in the warrior but the more tension created in the lats, the harder it is to permit the arms to lift up overhead since the natural tendency for the lats is to pull down the arms. A significant part of the skill of the performance of the posture is, thus, differentially relaxing the two parts of the same muscle. I cannot describe how this is done only that it needs to be done! The fact of this occurring when the posture is done" properly" leads one to master the posture –this takes many years. This process of differentially relaxing some structures is not peculiar to this posture but probably most difficult on this. To help understand the phenomenon what you can do is go into the first part of the posture with the legs in position and then hold the calf muscle of the forward leg and just wobble it around to make sure that it is not tight. It is common for practitioners to hold this muscle tight in the mistaken belief that the posture requires this –it does not as your test will instantly demonstrate. Practise the posture with this notion in mind, making deliberate relaxation of the calf muscle the early part of the postural set-up and attempt to keep this relaxation throughout the posture. When this can be done then at least the concept of differential relaxation—I will refer to this as DR---- will be intellectually understood if not fully acted upon.

The next difficulty of performing the posture is to allow the corset muscles many times referred to previously, to relax and take up the natural central position of trunk holding. The strong tendency during the performance of the warrior is for the trunk to rotate towards the rearward leg, partly as a result of corset tension, partly because of lack of experience and partly because of shortening down the hip flexor/ rectus femoris/hip joint structures and possibly shortening of psoas.

The effects of the posture are manifold, aside from that described above which can be considered as a benefit but is harder to classify. The principal benefit is strengthening of quadriceps at the front of the thigh— this produces static strength with elastic softness of muscle and not the hard strength of weight lifting. The posture aids circulation in lower limbs because of the temporary occlusion—blocking---of arterial and venous flow in the affected muscles. Holding the thigh muscle as contracted as it is possible to do—which means placing the thigh in the horizontal mode—will restrict blood flow but will increase blood pressure in the limb, partially affecting flow to the lower leg as well. This is achieved because of the presence of arteries passing down through the fascial clefts in the thigh muscles which when the muscle is held in tension will be squeezed hard, so creating a build up of pressure into the limb which is then relieved instantly by coming out of the posture. This phenomenon creates a flushing effect on all the poorly served blood vessels rather as a heavy downpour of rain would wash away old tree branches and rubbish contained in ditches. I believe this effect has significant benefits for those with a tendency to varicosing of veins. Varicose veins occur because blood has become static in the superficial veins, causing a collapse of the semi-lunar valves(these are one way

valves) —usually in legs but also anally as piles—and this may be the case because only the large vessels are working. If the small vessels in their thousands can be encouraged to do their share of blood transfer perhaps this would not occur. Of course, it has to be recognised as well that there are plenty of people with varicose veins whose parents had the same so genes must play some part.

The warrior performed " well" will lift the whole rib cage up and if it is performed with strongly held in breath it can aid the stretching of the abdominal myofascial structure to further expand the rib cage, bringing this part of the body closer to the child-like state.

The ankle will eventually be better flexed with this posture but this aspect is a feature of other postures as well.

Hip joints will obviously be stretched especially the ligaments binding the head of the femur, a common restrictor in Western culture, principally in extension which is not something that the vast majority of humans will be obliged to achieve.

However, it is better to consider that the warrior is not really done for stretching purposes, although some stretching will take place. Rather it is done to strengthen the will, to create greater understanding of differential relaxation—DR- and thus to free muscles to behave as they did in the child –like state which is with much more independence of action.

Reverse Triangle. Parivrtta Trikonsana
I have chosen this posture because for me it represents a " gold standard" in postural mastery. I do not like to use such a term as though once it " looks good" then it can be ticked off the list—but we do not have the language, as far as I am able to see, to describe another aspect. So I will explain what I mean. If I ask a group of yoga practitioners with which I have had no previous contact, to perform this posture, I watch for several

illuminating elements. The first is –who looks around the class to see how to do the posture. Second, who groans or complains or makes some other remark about the posture being difficult. Thirdly, how is it approached and finally what degree of spinal rotation takes place. Also I do watch to see if both legs are kept locked straight but the ultimate test is to observe if the posture is performed fully, that is to say, with full spinal rotation. To the benefits, then. The amount of spinal rotation is no different from that which takes place in the seated spinal twist—shall I say that this is so if" all other things are equal". But if a person has a full seated spinal twist but is not able to perform a full reverse triangle this requires investigation. The most likely cause is shortening of hamstrings.

The individual hamstring stretch in this posture is the finest available. Not only is the myofascial structure along the back of the thigh strongly pulled but also affected is the lumbar fascia on the opposite side of the pelvis/lumbar spine. In this respect it is a supplement to the seated spinal twist but probably more powerful. The posture is also a strong neck rotation but, of course, the neck is held in the horizontal position which it is not in the seated spinal twist.

The posture has the spine held horizontal which will be a spinal twist with abdominal organs suspended from the spine rather than under compression as in the seated spinal twist.

The posture is often performed with the lower hand placed on the outside of the forward foot. Whilst this may look good in a glossy book it is of little use to the average practitioner at the very least for the ten years it will take to get the maximum value out of the yoga process. It is, therefore, much more valuable to perform it with the feet and hand forming a broad base—and that is achieved with the floor hand placed at least 6 inches from the forward foot at the instep rather than on the outside of the foot. This will then allow the practitioner strong use of the hand on the floor to apply substantial leverage to create the maximum rotational force. This is the real value of the posture beyond other rotational postures—in this regard I would classify it as very powerful, much more so than seated spinal twist.

Whilst in the posture, it will be observed that the lower arm requires strong contraction of the same half of the trapezius muscle—but only half. Half of a muscle is seldom used—since we are creatures of habit it would be much more common for muscles to be used in distinct groups—this of course frequently uses much more energy than is really necessary. Part of the value of the posture is in the lesson it can give you –showing you how to relax that part of the body that does not need to be kept tense—another part of DR!—the spiritual benefit comes in this region; you learn how to genuinely let go and use only those muscles that is it is necessary to use. This itself is liberating from patterns of old behaviour. The posture provides fertile ground for self examination—how are you with the difficulty of performing this posture? Are you able to hold the posture still and concentrate upon the breath or an image, without the postural discomfort or muscular effort interfering with your quiet mind?. This aspect alone eventually permits you to " switch off"—this is not an accurate reflection of what is really meant. The use of the posture to assist in the focus upon something outside oneself—moving away mentally from the pain and difficulty inherent in performing the posture—is what enables the practitioner to gradually accept some of the principles being in the NOW. The focus upon one single thing permits the individual the unusual opportunity to just BE. No expectation, no boxes to tick, no person to satisfy, no hoops to jump through. Just being. The posture is being done just because it is—it has no objective, it has no purpose. When one can accept this and just do the postures with this attitude then yoga is well entrenched and the process of enlightenment is underway.

The hand and arm held aloft while the posture is performed is forgotten in the desire to fulfil the postural requirements. For the great majority of students of this posture, the hand is held in tension—this makes another part of the performance of much greater value than its simple expression would suggest!! Watch the tight hands and wrists during a workshop—and then instruct the students to allow the hands to be free and relaxed and observe that this in itself creates great difficulty. This is something else that provides food for the spiritual journey. Here once again the student is required to practice what I have called differential relaxation—let go of the hand tension but retain other tensions as needed to perform the posture.

Locust Posture. Salabhasana.
There are various interpretations of this posture so I will commence by saying that the posture in mind involves lying face down and raising arms and legs off the floor. The primary benefit is in the abdominal

compression created. There is no additional benefit over other posture of similar ilk when it comes to spinal muscle strengthening. There are several other postures as good as this for spinal muscle work.

The compression can be static and one can make the diaphragm work hard in this posture which can create a rocking motion which will create variation in the pressure. The overall benefit of this is to break down abdominal adhesions. The compression brings considerable changes to blood flow which itself means an increase in cell replacement rate and faster removal of toxic material. Most of the disorders under the modern umbrella term " diseases of consumption" can be classified by their lack of mobilisation of components of the body. In the ancient medical systems poor elimination is cited as one of the most serious causes of loss of health. Boat posture has a similar effect.

The Boat posture will enable the student to concentrate her mind on keeping still in this posture and just creating a strong focus for the mind. So aside from the physical benefits mentioned above, consider the most value from this posture to come from the mind and concentration opportunity created as result of doing something hard to hold for any more than a very short time.

Bow Posture. Dhanurasana.
This is conducted lying face down as in the locust but one grasps the ankles with the hands. Much the same comments can be made about this posture as were made about the boat but the back bending value is increased as a consequence of the ankle grasp although there is a good deal less extension of the spine takes place in comparison with the cobra. So it is best considered, once again, as a posture having mind calming potential and abdominal compression benefits. This posture probably also has more potential benefit in loosening the diaphragm if it has lost its mobility. For the very stiff athletic male, this will be a real issue and this posture should be worked at for a long time to gain the benefits of upper abdominal muscle loosening with its consequent additional benefit of better breathing resulting from the diaphragm being less fascially bound to the overlying muscles. Of course, this is a speculation based upon much observation and hands-on therapy with yoga follow up so it's a very well informed guess!

It is the alternate compression and decompression inflicted upon the abdominal contents that produces the strong inclination to reduce the adhesions between organs. In addition mechanical compression upon the intestines stimulates increases in the flow of blood and lymph as well as aiding peristaltic action, that mechanism which produces effective elimination from the bowels. In this posture all the organs hang away from the spine and especially the liver will be pressed directly and hard into the diaphragm making considerable increases in the pressure upon this organ. This alone will tend to soften the fascial coverings of the various organs. The fascial bags in which many of the abdominal organs are contained—these are called omentum and are of serous tissue so behave much like fascia and thus, in the state of immobility, can create adherence to the organ contained within and consequent interferences to lymph and blood flow.

Reclining Hero Posture.
Lying down between your own feet for many is seen immediately as impossible. It has to be admitted that for many men—almost exclusively men—impossible is what it is!!. But of course, it is only impossible now. The principal obstruction is always the shortening around the hip area, the ASIS again, which is usually the second most popular restrictor for the camel posture. The rectus femoris muscle, part of the quadricep group, attaches to the ASIS and creates a permanent limitor to the extension of the hip. The person cannot take the leg back behind the hip line. The typical physiotherapists solution to this shortening is to tell the person to grasp hold of the ankle and bend the knee fully, pulling the foot backwards to create the stretch. There is no question that the feeling of something stretching is created but it is far too weak a pull to have any effect except upon the softest of tissue. The very weak stretch on the rectus femoris clearly demonstrates the lack of real understanding in the profession as to what actually works. It is this bent knee method that is shown in books but it is nothing like as powerful a stretch as reclining hero which will be apparent within 10 seconds of attempting the posture!!

This posture, when the quadriceps are very tight, is extremely uncomfortable and will create low back pain. This results from the pelvis being tilted strongly which then makes the lumbar vertebrae press hard against one another. There is no harm here but it does create fear in some minds.

The primary value of the posture is in the strength of stretch in the quads—aside from that it is no different from lying down in corpse posture—but many times less pleasant!!

The fascial plane runs right down from the abdominal fascia, down the legs and along to the toes. It is possible to actually feel this whole fascial plane stretch when in the posture—but it takes a while before the pain of doing the posture has reduced sufficiently to allow you to feel something else except how difficult it is!! There is no other posture which can create this level of fascial stretch down the whole of the lower part of the body at the front. If you were to consider the forward bend and how this posture affects the whole of the fascial envelope along the posterior surfaces of the whole body then there is no direct equivalent for the frontal structures. This means the job of frontal stretching of the fascial envelope must be done in stages. The cobra, camel and reclining hero are the three principal elements of the alternative frontal stretch. Perhaps the wheel posture could be seen as a further piece of this jigsaw.

To augment this posture and to prove to yourself the fascial connection between parts of the body —especially those that you may feel cannot be connected—take the arms overhead after you have got yourself to be as low in the posture as possible. If this is very painful but you are lying on the ground then try the arms overhead and you should then feel the abdominal muscle fascia pulling right down the front of the thighs. So now you may be able to believe the old fashioned Deep South spiritual song—"your neck bone connected to your foot bone"" obviously to be sung to the correct tune!!!

If you now hold the arms overhead and breath in strongly so that the rib cage is lifted up and attempt to expand the ribs sideways at the same time, you will then have experienced the maximum potential of the posture.

Down Facing Dog. Adho.Mukha Svanasana.
Each yoga posture has some unique characteristic. For this posture I think it is the unique combination of partial inversion and strong stretching. There is another feature which makes this a particularly valuable posture and that is making the attempt to bring the spine to showing it's normal lordosis in the lumbar area. To do this requires the practitioner to push the chest towards the feet which in turn will increase the tension upon the hamstrings in a way not demanded in the —more

powerful –forward bend. One is required to use the hip flexors—namely the iliopsoas group—to bring the lumbar spine towards the feet thus increasing the tension upon the hamstrings. Needless to say the calf muscles—gastrocnemius and soleus—receive a good stretch. There is another position which can be attained which is far more effective upon calf muscles, however. In this posture the abdominal contents are allowed to fall onto the interior of the abdominal muscles and the diaphragm and away from the pelvic basin thus relieving congestive pressure upon all the viscera. Shoulder muscles are enabled to strengthen without too much demand at any one time. For those ===generally women—struggling to perfect the plank posture, the dog will move them towards this position quite quickly.

Breathing Practices.
We should consider some of these since these are vital in the production of spiritual effects. The mechanical effects are documented in yogic medical experiments of which there have been many BUT --and it is the same but as before, there is no explanation offered by the experimenters as to why the effects occur. Only WHAT is known. The rest is up for conjecture but my strong inclination is that the reason is the same as the Buddhist Dhammapada not citing any reasons for the mind working as it does.! It just is as it is because that is how it is! Fairly inadequate for any scientific mind!!.

Very unsatisfactory for those having a will to know more but the more one progresses in yoga the less inner demand exists for the reasons. The yogi is very contented to have found that which does actually work and happy to see that it is actually working on her just as it has for countless millions before. That has to be the only evidence worthy of note.

But let us nevertheless, proceed to see what happens. I propose to take kapalabhati, bhastrika and retained breathing mechanisms and state from published yogic medical trials what effects have been noted and any explanations which have been offered as to the reasons for such effects. Part of the reason for my writing this book has been to offer my opinions as to why things happen as they do since I have taught and thus observed a few thousand students of yoga in 25 years. I have also treated over 6,000 people during this time and have taught many to perform the postures that would be most effective in preventing a recurrence of their troubles. Necessarily, therefore, my observations are probably almost unique so I choose to offer these thoughts to any one interested simply because the scientific treatises offered by medical researchers offer little in the way of explanation. Perhaps they wish to leave the reader to make up their own conclusions but my experience of sitting for many hours in front of groups of students interested in the how and the why has obliged me to come up with rational explanations—but they are just that and not necessarily THE ABSOLUTE TRUTH.

The practices named above have been tested on many yoga students in many medical establishments in India. What has been examined has always been carbon dioxide and oxygen levels before and after the practices. If you consider this, it seems at first utterly inadequate but unavoidable since there is little else that science can MEASURE other than these two parameters. Various experiments on incarcerated persons have been conducted. Experienced yogis were put in an air tight cell with a known volume of oxygen and their breathing rate measured, along with oxygen and carbon dioxide consumption. The pattern to emerge in all these studies is that the experienced confined person consumes less oxygen than the normal person in the same circumstances. Now this cannot be explained by the breathing practices performed but can be explained by understanding mind control. When asked about the mind practices during the confinement the subjects claim to have " gone inside" and simply meditated. The same approximate characteristics occur during meditation so it reasonable to conclude that the oxygen/ carbon dioxide issue is quite irrelevant.

What can be demonstrated in the experiments is that during khumbaka, the retained breath phase of breathing practices, there is an increase in the oxygen content of the expelled air and a reduction in the " bad air" which can reasonably be explained by the following. Take a river as an example of fluid flow. Air is also a fluid and behaves just as does water. Water in a pipe behaves just as water in a river. In the centre of the pipe or river, flow is at its maximum whilst at the banks or surfaces of the pipe it is static or nearly static. Anyone can witness this standing by the banks of a river. All fluids behave in this way. Now, consider the inbreath and its passage through the bronchioles to the alveoli of the lungs. The air ways behave just as a river—the air up against the surface may not move –in quiet breathing it certainly is static like water in a slow flowing river. This means that the air against the airway may well be stale and not have been expelled for –perhaps—hours, especially if the person has been sitting and concentrating using a computer, shall we say. This dictates that the air in the alveoli may also be stale. Therefore, we take a strong and long inbreath during our practices and then hold this air for perhaps half a minute. All the stale air must then be diluted. The same phenomenon occurs if you pour a glass of water and then pour a thimble full of coloured juice into it —within a short time the whole water has become the colour of the juice. This is the same characteristic as occurs with air in the lungs.

The outcome of this process is that the diluted stale air is less stale when next you hold one full breath., This in turn is slightly less stale when the next in breath is taken and held. And so on—over a few minutes it is possible to cleanse all the air until there is virtually no stale air—this has certainly been measured as an increase in the oxygen content of expelled air. Now we can, I am sure, interpret this as beneficial especially when living in circumstances in which air is polluted by particulate matter. Any one living in a city matches this—diesel fuel is highly particulate, much like soot.

The kumbhaka phase does not exist in isolation and is part of a three or four part process. In this regard it is akin to imagining only performing one yoga posture---this is not likely to happen. Thus, dissecting this process and imagining one part to be of value is itself of limited use.

With this in mind, I turn to the in- breath and out- breath phase of the common yogic breathing practice. Firstly, it is usual to have performed a series of postures beforehand, thus making the individual more relaxed. The person has not been interrupted, no telephone or TV to interfere. So coming to the breathing practice now could create a reasoned argument that it is bound to have a beneficial effect!

You are sitting relaxed with the mind calm. You deliberately control the rate and force of the in-breath for a fixed quantity of seconds. You then hold the breath, perhaps with chin lock, and follow this with a controlled out-breath of, usually, twice the length of the in- breath. You demonstrate the ability to control your breath, making you well above the norm for your culture. You can learn to lengthen this breath which will enable you to slow down the rate of breathing which will have a reflex effect upon blood pressure and heart rate. The benefits of this are well known.

It is probable that the greatest benefit of this is spiritual or just plain mental. Stressed individuals who appear in my yoga classes show all the signs of this part of the process being the most valuable. Even the most impatient person when they get to this stage has slowed down and is not any longer in a rush to finish. There is a strong calming effect which should not be overlooked as having great significance.

Khapalabhati is strong abdominal contraction to expel air through the nostrils, repeated rapidly for several minutes. This involves a fast and rhythmic expulsion of air and passive in- breath, created entirely by recoil from rib intercostal muscles. This process sets up a low frequency vibration throughout the abdominal contents helping to break down adhesions between organs. Vibration has the effect of stimulating fluid flow but again there is a clear demonstration of control. Control of the breathing processes necessitates control of the mind. In all the breathing practices there is an immediate impact upon the nervous system. This aspect is covered later under the relevant title.

There is at first an increase in the oxygen content of the breath but this apparently stabilises and becomes normal, with some experimenters finding that there was a small reduction in oxygen content of the blood, indeed, and an increase in the carbon dioxide content. It is this notion that gives rise to experimenters believing that the overall benefit is in increasing the ability of the body to withstand increases in carbon dioxide—in other words to better tolerate pollution of the air. What yogic researchers have consistently done is to avoid conjecture and adhere firmly to scientific fact. I could put this last phrase in inverted commas!! This has been, largely, to avoid ridicule from members of the medical profession not willing to study yoga nor to consider it a scientific discipline. So that which I have placed in this book could come under the title—conjecture. But this means that all that is published is done with controlled trials on that which can be measured—and only that. There has been no allowance for the adepts opinion—indeed the experiments have been carried out upon those with no previous yoga experience so as to remove bias!. Also all experiments have been conducted using a range of postures and practices—never one practice. This makes any deductions of little value unless they are based upon the experience of many people. Thus, we return to conjecture based upon observation of many people since valuation of ones own practice is too small a sample to be credible in anyone's eyes.

Khapala bhati-----what occurs can best be described as the same effect as when wind is blowing over a body of water such as a lake and the wind suddenly ceases. There is a complete calm –and one can see through the water because the surface is no longer ruffled. This is the best way to describe the effect of this practice. The effect is immediate. It is a noted preparation for the business of meditation.

During the practice there are momentary increases in the pressure within the thoracic cavity and, attendant upon this is an increase in the blood pressure, causing a kind of pulsating effect, these pulses creating waves within the pipework of the vascular system. This would tend to expand and contract the elastic pipes removing kinks and minor obstructions., much like a hammer drill. Vibration is what breaks down hard surfaces.

This practice provides a valuable prelude to meditation. It is a preparatory practice and can be induced to create the quiet mind at any time, without the postural work beforehand if you so desire. It requires, for some people, weeks of attempting this to make it create the stated effect.

Bhastrika is performed by strong inhalation and exhalation. The word means bellows so the yogi performs a series of strong breathing movements with active in and out breath. Once again control has to be demonstrated. There is a large excursion of the diaphragm and thus a strong stimulus to all abdominal contents, with a similar impact upon organ function as that created by khapalabhati.

Both practices produce a serenity of mind after less than a minute of practice These are practices which create the correct mood for meditation. In this regard one might argue that the physical benefits are quite irrelevant since the vast majority of benefit in this area is already provided by the postures.

The mental benefits are immediately apparent to the new starter in yoga. It is always fascinating to watch new people in an established yoga class as there is usually some mild embarrassment which I assume is normal. The new persons facial expressions change immediately that breathing practices are encountered often resulting in extended periods of breathing practice beyond what any one else in the class is doing. In truth I do not know how to classify this characteristic except to place it under the spiritual banner.

The Healing Breath

This is usually the term given to the practice of breathing in, holding the breath and then controlling the outbreath. The ratio often used is breathing in to the count of 3, holding in for the count of 12—that is 4 times as long as the in breath—and then controlling the outbreath to the count of 6. Thus the ratio of 1;4;2 is established. This takes a good deal of practice before perfecting. The benefits are similar to other breathing practices and the variations possible are infinite. Once one has mastered the main mechanism then all manner of variations can be made.

The most immediate effect is mind-calming. The asthmatic/bronchitic is struck right away by her difficulty and then with practice, by the rate of improvement using this technique. In numerous scientific studies, the blood pressure, heart rate, blood sedimentation rate along with a host of other common medical indices of health, are recorded and the breathing practices are seen to be a vital part of the process of normalising the nervous system and glandular function.

14. The Spiritual Effects

It will not be difficult to see that this region of examination will not produce anything like the volume of detailed statistical or measured data produced by consideration of the purely physical postures. Of course this is because the researchers have almost universally been trying to prove the product to sceptical medical people. The reason for this—to try to dissuade medics to prescribe drugs when yoga would do the job much more effectively and at no cost. Whilst those reading this manual may well feel inclined to nod sagely and say something like" Well of course everyone would be better off if it were so"-----and so on. The reality is vastly different. In the next section I propose to set out just a few of the medical professions own statistics on patient harm and deaths created by medical intervention in all its forms—surgery, radiation and drugs. Or as the real cynics would say " cut, burn or poison".
For now let us consider what the spiritual changes are and where possible suggest the reason why they are created.

Entering the realm of yoga must be recognised as something of a starting point for all spiritual changes. Simply to enter the arena of yoga means that you are searching for something. If you keep it up for a few months—and especially if you practise at home—something has happened to you that cannot be explained in purely mechanical terms. If you were to ask colleagues at work to comment upon your appearance it is likely that they are at a loss to wonder why you are asking the question. Maybe this would alert them to considering that something is afoot!! But the question put bluntly" Can you notice any difference in my appearance?" the likelihood is that few would be able to say with hand on heart " oh yes, I see that you are _____ "

There is an old Zen saying " What do you do before enlightenment? Chop wood and carry water. What do you do after enlightenment? Chop wood and carry water!"

This strongly implies that one is the same after enlightenment as before—in appearance and physical activity. The enlightenment process, the journey to enlightenment, does not make one change into something different. It may well make you change occupation, go on a long pilgrimage, create the need to start another activity. What it does not do is fundamentally change your humanity. I am still going to be Andy Thomas, with the Virgo nature, still liking all sorts of music, still wishing to play my guitar and tend my garden. You are not going to be a different person to look at nor will there much change in your way of doing things. What will be vastly different will be what you discover about your own mind and how this helps you to live a more fulfilled life.

So---how does this come about? The greatest obstacle to a scientific analysis of this is that the spiritual change is that which occurs after the postural work and the pranayama. It may not be coincident with it so how would one be able to say that it is the postures or the breathing practices that have created the more enlightened state? Whereas, if you have a bad back and after 3 months of yoga your back feels much better and you have tried lots of treatment regimes which did not work, then surely you can scientifically state that the yoga postures have done the job. But---- even here you will have to accept that yoga is seldom entered into by those not seeking peace and calm and something that nothing else can give them. It may be that spiritual change is already like the seed, waiting in the soil for the best conditions for germination. How did the seed get there? Why you and not your friend and neighbour? Why so few people?

It is in this dark area that exists the most difficulty with scientific rationale.We are, thus, subject to debate and conjecture. The physical experiments conducted in yoga institutions using trained and untrained yogis, show clearly that chemical change takes place. Blood composition is different. Blood pressure reduces. Blood chemicals that are inappropriate in too great a quantity decline in quantity as a result of just performing the postures. These, again, are simple to measure and the people indulging in the experiments are trained to do as they are told and not to do anything else that would affect the results. The participants in the experiments are requested to sign a contract to state that they will comply with the carefully documented requirements of the experiments. The postures to be performed have to be carried out in accord with a properly designed programme. Nothing is left to chance. So we can reasonably conclude that no spiritual change will take place in this experiment. Even if it did, it is very unlikely that those in charge of the research would be interested to hear about it because it is not what they are measuring. Once again, then, we return to conjecture and we must be willing to accept that people generally enter the realm of yoga because of some deep spiritual need, the nature of which they may well not comprehend. I am fairly certain, as a result of many discussions with yoga students over many years, that there is a point, almost a EUREKA moment, at which they " get it"—this may well be the first ball to roll in the pin ball machine of the process!! How it begins to roll cannot be known. How it is that some can be literally kicked up against the machine many times and still avoid entering the realm of the spiritual journey.? It cannot be known.

Buddhists have a simple explanation for this. They say that the vast majority of people in the world are of " limited scope" whilst a small minority are of " intermediate scope" and the microscopic quantity are of " advanced scope". This is a very easy concept to understand. It makes no judgements. It is a plain simple statement of fact, as they see it. It certainly makes comprehension very plain as well—it just is like it is!! They offer no reason. It is one of the very great simplicities of Buddhism—there is no attempt to explain why-- it is just an observation of what is. Likewise within the Buddhist precepts, what is written in the Dhammapada, the Way of Moral Truth, is that the mind is flighty and fickle and flies after its fancies whenever it can. There is no attempt anywhere in this text so say WHY the mind works as it does. It is so and that is the end of it. Indeed, here am I saying this but even this is not said in one of the most famous works of philosophy—there is no statement like"" it is like this but we don't know why". You may say it would be good to have had such a statement-but it is not there. Neither is such a statement in anything written by Patanjali---it is certainly not in the Sutras.

Yogis have, thus, been restricted to stating that which they have found to work—without conjecture. Mine is a book full of conjecture. There is none in ancient works of yoga philosophy. A further conjecture on my part is that there is a very simple reason for this. If you want to receive peace and compassion and love as part of your daily life, just do it. Take up yoga. Do it. Don't intellectualise about it. Don't analyse the reasons, just get on with it. If you consider what most people who come to yoga do it is exactly this. They simply turn up and follow the path similar to that taken by a religious mendicant-just follow the path and it will lead to enlightenment.

This makes our search for WHY even harder to justify as well as more difficult to achieve. I propose to start with an analogy. Most people, I believe, are in a sort of jungle of life, a place of confusion. We no longer have a tribal leader who would lead us to where the tribe ought to go. Indeed, there are no longer any wise ancients to move the tribe spiritually. At least, they are not visible as they would have been within a tribal scenario. We have Government and religious leaders and politicians but no spiritual leaders.

Coming to yoga is part of the deep search, usually created by an inner demand and appealing to a small minority. They do not usually know what it is that they seek but know what it is that they do not want. The presence of silence and stillness creates an internal realisation that these are the circumstances in which much resolving of internal issues of distress can be laid to rest. Nothing else gives them this feeling—it appears that performing the postures creates a sort of permanent state of calmness and stillness. Their aches and pains decline. Their fears decline. They feel more aware, more alert. If they have kept up practise then after about 6 months it has become plain that there is a significant change in personal well being. If you ask the question of each person "how has it happened"? they do not know, only that they feel better and then can tell you that change has taken place. If you say Why ? the answer is always because I have been doing yoga. So no matter where one looks there is never a why only a what.

The why has to remain conjecture. And it has to remain unmeasured and general. More blood flow, more lymph flow. Of course, this book represents my attempt to explain why it should be undertaken!!

We can ask the same question of most things that happen in the World, can we not\? Why does the earth revolve? Why is gravity necessary? It simply is as it is and human life could not be visualised any other way, so say many writers on the subject. How could human life be imagined without love, without food, without water---we define human life as being dependent upon these things. Acceptance of all elements of humanity is necessary in order just to be able to see the normal human condition.

15. Effects upon the Nervous System.

Since there is very regularly confusion about the meaning of this system I propose to include a brief resume of what constitutes this system

The Central Nervous System—the CNS—consists of brain, spinal cord 12 pairs of cranial nerves which do not emerge from the spine and 31 pairs of spinal nerves. These nerves give off branches to various organs and tissues. The nerve trunks and their branches constitute what is known as the Peripheral Nervous System. The brain and spinal cord are large masses of nerve cells, their processes and neuroglia cells. The spinal cord is a prolongation of the brain and is composed of grey and white matter, the grey being nerve cells and the white nerve fibres. These latter elements are the processes or axons of the nerve cells. Within the brain grey matter forms the outer part and the white matter lies inside whilst in the spinal cord the reverse is the case. Nerves are thread –like structures made of fibres with an outer connective tissue covering. Some nerves consist mainly of motor nerve fibres and are called motor or efferent nerves which carry the orders from the nerve centre to the organ for action—usually a muscle. The second type consists of sensory nerve fibres and are known as sensory or afferent nerves which carry information to the brain. The ending of the sensory nerve is called the receptor which receives the stimulus.

Generally there are two types of nerve impulse which form the basis of any nervous function—1. inhibitory impulse which starts the process of inhibition or stopping of a function and 2. acceleratory or excitatory which starts a function.

The cerebrum is the physical basis of the mind with two cerebral hemispheres, right and left. The cerebral cortex has motor and sensory areas forming the outer part of the cerebrum. In man the cerebral cortex is highly developed and is considered the highest part of the nervous system regulating all functions of the organism by linking the body with the external environment.

The cerebellum is located behind the medulla oblongata and pons and below the posterior side of the cerebrum. The cerebellum is well connected with the cerebrum, pons, medulla oblongata and other parts of the brain. Activities of the cerebellum are of a reflex character. Though the voluntary movements are initiated by the cerebral cortex, their efficient performance depends upon the cerebellum. The cerebellum is engaged in co-ordination, distinctiveness and smoothness of movements. It also predicts the future course of movement with the help of the cerebrum and maintains the muscle tone. It is involved in body balance, running, dancing, speech and walking.

The medulla oblongata and the pons constitute the brain stem. It contains the network of nerve cells and nerve cells and fibres and it is engaged in reflex function and conduction of ascending and descending impulses. It contains vitally important centres of cardiac activity—respiration, vasomotor activity, digestive activity, defence reflex like coughing and vomiting

The hypothalamus is an important centre of the autonomic nervous system to regulate many activities such as metabolism, heat production, pituitary function, arterial blood pressure, heart activity. It is also engaged in emotional effects through the autonomic nervous system.

The nerve fibres are grouped in tracts or nervous pathways. Some tracts are descending—these are motor nerves—and some are ascending—these are sensory. Motor and sensory merge with each other and form the spinal nerve root. A pair of spinal nerves emerges between the two vertebrae.

The main activity of the spinal cord is conduction of nerve impulse and reflex activity. Muscle tone is maintained by the reflex action. Proprioceptors like muscle spindles, tendon organs when stimulated due to changes in position of muscles, send impulses to the spinal cord.

Autonomic—sympathetic and parasympathetic.
These are the names given to those aspects of the human nervous system that—very broadly—stimulate and then quieten. The sympathetic system tends to make everything get going and the parasympathetic slows it all down again, bringing the whole body back to what we could call a point of homeostasis. The sympathetic dilates the pupils, decreases the secretion of saliva and tears, constricts the small arteries but dilates the coronary arteries and elevates blood pressure. The parasympathetic system roughly, brings it all back to "normal". We could use the word equilibrium but many writers choose to avoid this word stating that there is never a point at which the human being is static. Homeostasis is the word applied to the state of balance which is constantly being worked on by these two parts of the autonomic nervous system. So we could use the term dynamic balance, implying a constant state of maintenance. Broadly, the sympathetic makes secretions for digestion and stimulates the digestive processes while the parasympathetic system would calm the whole process down once eating had taken place. These two systems affect all glandular functions and all abdominal organ functions. The nerve pathways--- we might call it the hard wiring of the systems --- are universally covered in living tissues unlike electrical cables, and thus the quality of stimulus carried by the nerve fibres is dependent upon the quality of lymph and blood flow to all the tissues. Direct compression upon nerve trunks is known to affect the quality of flow of signals and has given rise to the widespread use of the words "trapped nerve" as a catch-all for pains felt around the spine! Of course, what direct compression does is to impede the flow of arterial blood to the coverings of the nerve trunks and associated structures.

What is well known in yoga is that sympathetic and parasympathetic activity is "normalised" by the practices of yoga and the probable explanation is, once again, the improvement of blood and lymph flow, with cellular repair rate improving.

If we conclude this to be the case—that is to say, if we collectively agree that this is the most likely mechanism, then it is not difficult to make the leap of faith to the position that the primary effect of yoga is improvements in blood and lymph with consequent increases in cellular repair rate. Thus we could equally easily conclude that it is the act of interference to cellular repair rate that creates all that we largely label the " ageing process". It may be that this is the real explanation for the many references to yoga making the yogi able to live forever or remove the ageing process. !! Another pure speculation.

In major works of neurology—medical text books—there is no attempt to locate the cause of any of the diseases of the nervous system. There are frequent references to diseases of parts of the brain and central/autonomic nervous system but a total absence of any explanation for the cause. There is a similar lack of substance in books on pathology. There are always lists of all the viral, bacterial or degenerative conditions and their effects but these are as usual, not accompanied by any structural allusions. No statement can be found to suggest that compression or degeneration with age causes a certain condition except in the obvious conditions such as Alzheimers or motor neuron disease. There are, equally, no references in medical text books, to the effects of compression of nerve roots or trunks—with the exception of Dr Cyriax, of course. A genuine lone voice. His statements on this issue largely revolve around the instigation of parasthesia, which is the medical term for change of sensation. Tingling and numbness are two of the most noted characteristics of nerve compression.

What is also of great interest is that there is no reference in any of the medical text books I have read, to suggest that what one eats has any effect upon the pathological condition !

In a paper written by Sarada Subrahamanyam a founder member of the VHSMedical Centre in Madras, entitled Yoga and Psychosomatic Illness, there is an interesting dissection of the workings of the nervous system. I will reproduce it here

". The neuromuscular or motor part of the nervous system has two parts known as tonic and phasic. Of these the phasic is most obvious since it involves the stimulus to movement. It is the tonic which forms the background to the ability of the phasic to function and it is the tonic part which does not impinge upon the conscious. In general the exteroceptive impulses excite the phasic reactions(which are transitory) while the interoceptive impulses regulate the tonic reactions. It is important to realise that while the phasic movement is momentary, involving a group of muscles, the interoceptive-tonic mechanism is continuous and diffuse and provides at all times the means by which phasic movements are possible. It is obvious that the " postural substrate" in a normal organism is and has to be in a continuously dynamic and fluid state, varying with the demand made on the body or mind, in order to provide an ideal background for any action contemplated. What is not so obvious is that the elasticity of this extremely malleable " substrate" can, under conditions of stress and disease, be strained to the limit. Yoga teaches that by attacking the abnormal postural substrate and reconditioning it to its previous adaptable and dynamic state, modifications of the emotional state can be obtained, leading to a state of mental tranquillity."

Probably this is the best synopsis I have read. It makes it clear that stress will create an abnormal state of muscle tone and it is this that will be most affected by mental calming.

16 The Confusion of the Modern

I have termed the phrase The Stupidity Conspiracy to describe that phenomenon which has created a medical system which has no interest in discovery of causes, which happily hands out death-creating pills, cheerfully dismisses mass death creation as part of every day life and constantly is subjected to assaults from outside from those who are sharply critical of the quantity of cash the system absorbs and shows no signs of needing less.

This term comes from the feeling that I used to harbour within myself, based upon early failure at school and the feeling that resulted from this experience, which I refer to now as a belief of my own stupidity. When I started in osteopathic practice in the early 1980's, it caused me a good deal of consternation when patients came reporting that they had numerous treatments from MR XXXXX who I considered to be a God amongst professionals. My early fumblings fairly quickly turned to a realisation that there were many unhappy people out there, who had spent their own money badly. I felt at first as if there must be a conspiracy of silence amongst the best of the health professionals—they all knew that I was stupid and all that happened was designed to permit me further food to keep this idea alive. A form of self-delusion. I felt as if there could be no possibility of me being able to restore patients already seen by really clever people who had failed. It must be me who is truly stupid and self-delusional. The term The Stupidity Conspiracy seems to conjure up very well what this feeling was even though the name has only just come to me during the writing of this book.

Here is my latest current example. Surely Pilates must be a very clever system designed by people cleverer than the yogis, otherwise surely it would not be preferred to such an ancient system.? This thought has echoed around my skull for a few months thus stimulating several discussions with those involved in it. When we come to the issue of core stability I simply ask—" what does this mean". The replies are varied but nebulous and inexact. " Well, it is a matter of keeping the spine stable" is one. " You want to strengthen the core muscles" says another. " What are the core muscles" I ask. The reply has been varied but the theme seems to be that the core is about the abdominal muscles. I am confused as to what the term core really means when the word in the dictionary means deep within. The abdominal muscles are external not internal. The internal deep muscles could be referred to as psoas and iliacus—but how has it been possible for someone to tell if these needed strengthening—I have not found more than a couple of patients in 25 years whose psoas was genuinely weak, as opposed to simply neurologically interfered with. If it has been then neurological disease would be the probable cause. What is meant by stability—the dictionary suggests lack of movement— isn't this the exact opposite of what yoga is trying to do?? But unfortunately, Mr Pilates has borrowed quite a lot from yoga and bashed it about a lot. He has used the plough posture dynamically and repeatedly –but why? What is the point of this method of using the posture? The plough has a strong value as a stretching posture for the upper muscles especially trapezius—how will this take place if the movement is undertaken without stopping for the stretch to take place? None of this sort of question can be answered by the system because it has not evolved as yoga has, over thousands of years. The fact that there is no underpinning philosophy in Pilates makes it just another exercise—but it seems to have gripped people. The only rational explanation for the grip is that there are few of them thinking about what is actually being asked of them—which mirrors the culture generally. This seems to bring us right back to the conspiracy—is it just that I cannot see it –or is there really a great deal of stupidity around?

Perhaps I can leave this part with a quotation from Albert Einstein
" Of two things I am fairly certain. One is the vastness of the Universe
and the other is the extent of human stupidity. I am just not SURE about
the former". Perhaps the drug industry is the mirror upon a society of unthinking people.

Much of what happens today can only be explained by my assertion that
there is very little original thinking happening. In yoga and therapy there
is a great deal of repetition of a formula. This is confirmed by several
NHS physiotherapists recently presenting for treatment.

17. Control. Self-Discipline.

Just a very superficial examination of the daily life of the average person
will show that there is little need for demonstrations of self-control, other
than the plain and simple. You are required to avoid driving over anyone
and you do have to get up and go to work. These are the simple
straightforward daily demands made upon the vast majority but I am
alluding to something way beyond the mundane. The person attending
karate lessons each week or playing a musical instrument is moving
closer. The person simply playing a musical instrument purely for
pleasure but, entirely of their own volition, teaching themselves how to
play more pieces or to improve technique, demonstrates the sort of self-
discipline that I refer to. In this way the daily practice of yoga or tai chi or
some other type of self-motivational discipline puts the individual into a
category where they will constantly be required to show CONTROL. I
use the term self-discipline because it is well understood. But actually I
prefer to use the word control because this is a further development of
the same characteristic. Let 's take an example. The breathing practice
earlier referred to as the healing breath—breathing in for the count of 3,
holding the breath for the count of 12 and then exhaling to the count of
6, is patently an exercise in control. Once one recognises this then the
notion of it doing good by changing the oxygen balance or cleaning the
lungs, can so easily just be taken for granted. The benefits to the
physiology can be fully accepted and acknowledged whilst much more
strongly orienting oneself around the concept of improving the quality of
control. The better the quality of control the better will be the
physiological benefits and the less one will even consider them. This
aspect has not, as far as I have read in all the yogic medical literature,

been mentioned except in passing. For me this is vastly more important and this is so, in my view, because we have lost, in our culture, all the requirements for self-discipline that would have been a natural part of living. Before the advent of the car and the phone and the computer, life would have demanded for all the self-discipline of self-transportation, fire lighting to keep warm, growing your own veg. The needs were constant and this may explain why only the tough survived. This was more akin to the animal kingdom in which, if you have a fault, you will almost certainly be killed as a weak member of the herd. Today there is very little such demand left and it may explain the rise of gymnasia –it may also explain the rise of the numbers attending yoga and tai chi.

Whilst this treatise is solely about yoga I have made a couple of references to tai chi and this is because it is a discipline that I have performed daily for the last 20 years and have taught for about 10 year. It has very little physical connection to yoga but a great deal in the self-discipline department. It is much harder to learn than is yoga and whilst I have taught many thousands of people to perform yoga postures, in a similar time I have not taught more than about 30 people tai chi. This is because the level of difficulty and the self-discipline required is much too great for most people. It takes years to learn a tai chi form well enough to perform it without a teachers correction. It takes another 10 years to perfect it with daily work—yoga is easy in comparison and instantly effective whereas tai chi may well only give you pain and mental torture for many years.!!

Control of the breathing rhythms demonstrates a level of self-control which, when allied to meditation, will enable the individual to separate themselves from the minds prattling. It is via the self-control of breathing that it can be easily demonstrated how the mind can be corralled by constant practice. In this regard it could be argued that the posture contributes little to this aspect of human behaviour.

18. Yogic Philosophy. Yamas and Niyamas

I cannot finish this book without just some reference to the underpinning ethical structure of the process since we are looking at how and why it works. The how and the why cannot simply be explained by the physical practices. In my 20 years of yoga teaching I have witnessed some practising yoga who exhibit very little awareness of the process and very little of what could be called spirituality. I have concluded that the reason for this is that they have simply indulged in the physical practices and have not found the need to examine the philosophy. The study of the ethical foundation of yoga is a requirement stated numerous times in the ancient texts and one can see why this is from the above example. If you want to journey along the spiritual path at least some understanding of the ethical foundation of life itself would be helpful.

I do not propose to examine all the yamas and niyamas here but do wish to highlight some of the elements for examination.

If we were to take santosha –contentment—you might be inclined to say that you are not contented or could be if only you had_____(whatever it is that you feel is missing) then life would be fine. Santosha is really a way of explaining that one needs to practice BEING contented, one needs to actually make an effort to be contented by fully and deeply examining the reasons why one states a lack of such. The postures provide the ideal opportunity to achieve contentment because they are outside of normal life and are the easy place to begin the process of becoming contented. We can use an example that I regularly employ in my classes. Take the reverse triangle posture which is one in which most people have difficulty and many express their frustration at not being able to make it perfect. How, then, can you be content with this posture if it is done less well than the teacher is demonstrating? First we can examine the origin of this discontent. Is this part of the programme given to you by the culture, by parents, by school or those at work? It is common today for young people to be " motivated" by teachers to do better by goading them into self-improvement. Were you given a " could do better" script? Are you never satisfied because you don't ever finish anything to your satisfaction? Is this because what you do is not ever done well or is it because you do not give yourself enough time to make it well done? These are the sort of questions to ask of yourself in order that you can approach the posture that is difficult, with equanimity. Do the posture with the attitude of " no mind". Just do it and do not allow any mental activity to take place, especially anything negative. Complete the posture to the best of your ability and then when you come out of the posture do not allow any comment to be made about the quality of the posture nor permit yourself to look at how it has been done by any one else. This mental position can gradually be brought to the point at which you can actually state to yourself that you are doing the posture and being content with how it is at the moment. This does not produce the state of complacency as has been suggested by some people. It simply removes the pressure to conform that is deeply rooted in our society. In this way one produces the state of contentment simply because the work in the posture gradually brings the practitioner to the expert stage in which her posture is indeed very good.

If we turn our attention to the issue of ahimsa, literally interpreted as non-violence, it is through the understanding of the true meaning of this that one can begin to change ones own mind-set. And it is, perhaps, in this area that most improvements can be seen to be resulting from the act of taking up yoga. Non –violence takes one into the realm of self-harming. Not just the physical but the mental as well. Performing a posture badly and then allowing yourself to be highly self-critical is an example of violence to the self. Stating negative comments about others is violence. Thinking violent thoughts is the same. It is, therefore, in this area of spiritual ethics that the true gains from yoga can come about. Best if one can combine an understanding of the need to " open out to all lifes possibilities" whilst engaged in performing the cobra posture or the camel.

19. Concluding Remarks

Have I met the objective, to explain how and why yoga works?. The how of yoga has been easy to explain. I still wrestle with the why. It is because it is not answerable in the same manner or extent. Indeed, the why can be reasonably answered as follows—Why does it work? Because it just does!!

We are not able to say why things work as they do. Why does sound not travel through a vacuum? Why is light refracted by a prism? There are a million things we cannot answer—we can say what happens and the mechanism—the how. We don't know why it is ordered to be so since we could assume that it could be ordered differently.

Why do we have 5 toes and not 6 –or 4—is five an important number? From an articulatory perspective it does not matter—we could function well with either

What we can say about the disease process is that poor nutrition will be demonstrably effective in reducing the person to a less well state. We can say that if one drinks foul water, there will be likely some disease. If sleep is deprived there will be an outcome. If you are hit be a car there will be some tissue injury. These are easy states to direct attention to. But for the vast majority there is no obvious evidence of events leading up to disorder. There is just TIME. This dictates to the shallow thinker that time equates with age—so that one declines with age and this is the usual extent of thinking. Whilst there is inevitably some loss of cell repair rate with passage through the age of 25, it is not linear and it not universally the same speed. There are many people of my age—currently 63—who would say that they are not doing anything like as much as they did when they were younger. In my case, I can still climb a tree, swing from a branch and run as fast as I could when I was young—er!! Other than the obvious wrinkles there is no loss of muscle tone and no increase in weight. There is no loss of function and I can do all the things that I could do when I was 18. This is not genetic disposition since my parents had a whole host of diseases and disorders and gradually shrunk into oblivion. They were constantly in and out of doctors surgeries and hospitals. This has not been my life at all and it shows no sign of changing. For me, age is just a concept.

Yoga is for those pursuing a spiritual journey. It does not attract others. It has its greatest appeal to what I refer to as the Socratean inquisitiveness. This is not for its own sake. This is not so that the process can be justified. It is simply that curiosity is part of the make up of a few people—so it really is for these few that I write this book, knowing perfectly well that this will be uninteresting to anyone else. If you are thirsty, I hope that this potion slakes your thirst.

I wish to conclude with a lovely quote from Albert Einstein
" Great spirits have always encountered violent opposition from mediocre minds"
There is another equally wonderful;
"For those who do not believe no proof is possible. For those who do believe, no proof is necessary"

Perhaps that is the real answer.

But I feel, having just discovered this in a book written about the life of Ida Rolf, the instigator of Rolfing, that the last word should be with her; "I don't know WHY it works, I only know THAT it works. I invent all these explanatory rationalizations later on"

Rolf,I. 1960. *Ida Rolf Talks*
Colorado, Boulder Press

Sounds familiar.

***

Andy Thomas. Nottingham, UK. 2008. Copyright protected. Intellectual Property Rights established. The author claims rights to protect this information but will happily enter into correspondent with anyone wanting to use this data for the benefit of humanity.

Lightning Source UK Ltd.
Milton Keynes UK
18 May 2010

154359UK00001B/102/P